iatrogenesis

iatrogenesis

Essays on Becoming a Physician

University of Michigan
Medical Students

iatrogenesis

Book design: Kevin Woodland, Publishing Services
Health Information Technology & Services
Michigan Medicine

Cover photo: Stephanie Owyang, Student
University of Michigan Medical School
Reprinted with permission

Produced by Publishing Services
Health Information Technology & Services
Michigan Medicine

Published by Michigan Publishing
University of Michigan Library

Names within essays have been changed
to preserve confidentiality.

ISBN: 978-1-60785-481-4 (softcover)
ISBN: 978-1-60785-482-1 (electronic)

Dedication

This book is dedicated to all
medical students—past, present, and future.

Contents

Foreword

In 2003, the University of Michigan Medical School developed a course for medical students known as the Family Centered Experience (FCE). I was privileged to teach the course for 15 years, from its inception to the final class. That experience has undoubtedly been the most memorable and meaningful period in my long career as a physician-educator.

FCE engaged students in the personal side of medicine through firsthand encounters with patients and their families. Medical students visited, in their homes, patient volunteers who had chronic or life-limiting illnesses. The volunteers discussed topics with the students such as how illness impacts one's sense of self or how they reacted to receiving life-changing health news. Following each home visit, the students wrote narratives reflecting on chronic illness and humanistic doctoring in light of their conversations with the volunteers. These essays illuminated the perspectives of the students: youthful coming-of-age narratives on the road to becoming physicians. The students' essays brought to life pitfalls, perils, and misadventures as they learned from patients, families, nurses, doctors, and certainly from each other. Reading these essays, I could feel their growing desire to see life with another's perspective, the development of empathy and compassion while striving for competency, and the yearning for graduation day and the open door to residency.

I imagined that a book composed of student essays charting the course of the four years of medical school could offer insight into this journey. I discussed the idea with a medical education colleague, Dr. Heather Burrows, and together we agreed to assess whether a critical mass of students might be interested in this project. The student body responded with overwhelming support and enthusiasm. Student writers volunteered and a student editorial group was formed. It became a fully student-driven project. It became a book.

Dr. Burrows and I are immeasurably proud of these students. It is their work which follows.

Andrew R. Barnosky, DO, MPH
Professor of Emergency Medicine and Anatomy
University of Michigan Medical School
Michigan Medicine

Foreword

Over 25 years after starting medical school, I still find myself swapping stories of my student experiences with other physicians. When Dr. Barnosky reached out to me with the idea for this book, I was thrilled at the chance to share the experience of medical training with others. My medical school years were full of moments that changed my perspective on the world around me.

As a child from a non-medical family, the world of medical school—from dissecting a cadaver to being present for the birth of a baby to sharing life-changing news with patients and families—was entirely foreign to me. Almost every day led to further discoveries of what it would mean to be a doctor. Just as I was fascinated by learning what was going on inside my body, I was also learning about the joys and struggles of the doctors around me. My classmates and I discovered the challenge of balancing the systematic thought processes of clinical medicine with the warmth and compassion that is fundamental to patient care.

Over the years, I have continued to reflect on those experiences and further understand the transformation I went through in the process of becoming a doctor. Although the field of medicine is constantly changing, medical students are still going through many of the same crucial moments I did and contemplating the impact medicine will have upon their lives. It has been tremendously exciting to see this book come to life. I hope that you share in the wonder as these students take you along on their journeys through medical education.

Heather L. Burrows, MD, PhD
Associate Professor of Pediatrics and Communicable Diseases
University of Michigan Medical School
Michigan Medicine

Prologue

"We forget all too soon the things we thought we'd never forget."
– Joan Didion
Slouching Towards Bethlehem

———————

Joan Didion wrote this in "On Keeping a Notebook," an essay to which I am partial because I too have kept some form of journal since I was a child. I am partial to Didion because her essay, "On Leaving New York," so closely mirrored my own experience leaving that city that it brought me to tears while cuddled into the window seat of a 737 destined for Ann Arbor, Michigan and the start of medical school. And, I am partial to this quote because it is, in fact, the impetus behind this very collection.

There was a morning during my third-year clinical rotations when I sat at a computer with a medical chart open, but instead of familiarizing myself with the patient's problems, I counted the days on the calendar. When the intern sat down next to me, I introduced myself. "I'm Katherine, the medical student who will be working with you in clinic today."

The intern grunted a hello and asked me how many rotations I had completed.

"I'm in the middle of third year. Break is coming up and I can't wait," I said. "Everything has become exhausting the last few weeks. But I bet you remember that feeling." I was sure he would remember just how hard it was to be a medical student, when you know so little and seemingly everyone, including yourself, expects you to know so much.

"No, actually, I don't," he replied. "I've forgotten most things about medical school."

His glib remark made me shirk, and his flat tone made me sad. For despite being in need of a break, the six months I had spent learning medicine hands-on had utterly wowed me. I wondered how this intern could forget the power (and the fear) he felt upon realizing he could ask a patient literally any question, and that he would receive an answer. I wondered how he could forget the surreal feeling, as if someone had just left the room, when a patient was pronounced dead. I wondered how he could forget first noticing the quickening pace of a patient's breath as she became septic, or the miraculous improvement of a febrile child when he received antibiotics. I wondered if I, too, would forget these things; a worry that has left me with several notebooks half-filled with lab results, rounding notes, and scenes much like those contained in these essays.

I read the essays submitted for this collection during my final semester of medical school. I had all but graduated save two pieces of paper—the envelope containing my residency placement, and my medical school diploma. I was surprised by how, while each essay was written by a different author capturing a unique moment, the essays together told a story of a doctor's development—a story not unlike my own.

I too remember, as a first year, the astonishment I felt for having lived in my body for nearly a quarter-century without understanding how it works. I too remember, as a second year, the discomfort I felt during a psychiatry lecture on schizophrenia and its seemingly hopeless prognosis, for sitting next to me was a friend whose brother had been diagnosed with the disease a year prior. I too remember, as a third year, the realization that a career other than medicine might have been equally fulfilling. And as a fourth year, I shared with my peers a growing reverence for the fragility of our bodies and the capriciousness of life. The stories in this collection resonated with me and the arc of my own narrative as a medical student. That they do speaks to the universality of one's maturation in becoming a doctor, and to the potency of this collection.

Medical school, to me, has always felt like a second childhood. We entered this world as innocents, beloved and adored by parents and professors who beam at us, remind us of how we are special, and swaddle us in white cloth. Everything in the world of medicine is new, and we are invited to touch, smell, see, and listen—to explore the human body to the utmost. Curiosity and observation are skills perfected by children, and by physicians, too. Donning a white coat and a stethoscope feels at first like playing dress-up. Hearing a heart murmur, like the thrill of learning how to tie one's shoes. Closing an incision, like riding a bike. While medical school is full of study, it is also full of play. The hospital is ours in a way that it is no one else's.

And like children, we as medical students soon learn that within our wondrous world is ugliness; within our perfect selves, fault. There is a sadness and disappointment that accompanies this disillusionment, and a beauty in the meaning we learn to make of it.

Once, while standing in the trauma bay, watching the doctors and surgeons resuscitate a 19-year-old who had been badly injured in a motorcycle crash, my eyes drifted up towards the ceiling and my mind to the ten floors beyond. I stood in awe of the singular dramas unfolding in the rooms before and above me. There had been a point in my life, not long before that moment, when I had never known about this place and all the stories, including my own, that it held. How could I not have known? How could I ever forget this feeling, right now?

Katherine Bakke
On behalf of the Editorial Board

Acknowledgments

We offer our thanks, first and foremost, to the authors featured in this collection who have generously shared stories, both intimate and honest, in order to illuminate the joyous and fraught process of becoming a physician. Without their words, this collection would not be possible.

Thanks also to the editors who have been fundamental in bringing this book to life with their collective passion for clear writing and strong editing. We are grateful not only for the editorial board's dedication to this project, which took two years to complete, but also for the friendships forged because of it.

We are indebted to Dr. Barnosky and Dr. Burrows, whose vision enabled the creation of this book. Our appreciation for your commitment to medical students and to honoring our experiences cannot be overstated. We are fortunate to have worked on this project with you both as our mentors.

We thank Publishing Services, part of Health Information Technology & Services at Michigan Medicine, for their assistance and expertise in making this collection something you can hold in your hands. Thanks to medical students Michael Dieterle and Gina Yu for their design ideas.

Thanks also to the Office of Medical Student Education and its M-Home Educational Enrichment Pillar. We especially thank Jennifer Hebestreit and Robert Cermak for supporting the efforts of students outside the lecture halls and the wards and for imagining a broader scope for medical student education. The M-Home initiative and our medical school family are what have made our experience at the University of Michigan Medical School truly unique.

Finally, we would like to thank the University of Michigan Medical School faculty, its residents, our fellow students, and, most importantly, our patients. Names within essays have been changed to preserve confidentiality. These are the people who urge us to constantly consider what it means to be good physicians and inspire us to do better each and every day.

And thank you, of course, to our families and friends. The process of becoming a physician is a singular one, but it cannot be journeyed alone. For accompanying us on this path, we are infinitely grateful.

Katherine Bakke, Whit Froehlich, and Trisha Paul
Editorial Board Leadership

Pre-Clinical Essays

Heart Sounds

Anita Vasudevan

My foundation for understanding health, healing, and medicine was laid by a well-intentioned bribe: at three years old, I was promised I could have the Sesame Street doctor play-kit I had been ogling for weeks at Toys-R-Us if I got potty-trained. Two weeks later, I was convinced I could cure my grandma's migraines by running up to her room with my Big Bird-embossed doctoring bag and gently rubbing her forehead. Looking back, this moment still holds for me what I believe to be the very essence of practicing medicine: being present with patients in times of pain, change, and illness.

Donning my first-ever white coat at the ceremony that marked the beginning of our medical training, I did not think I would end up spending the months after wondering if I had chosen a path that truly resonated with my beliefs. I had expected medical school to be the place where I would finally be able to learn how to be with people at their most vulnerable and to bring forth their humanity, and my own, in times of illness. I had expected to learn how to translate stories of challenges in health into action plans for empowerment and healing. But the first year of medical school has been something entirely different.

Instead of learning how to care for and about people, I spend my days as a pre-clinical student memorizing what seems like an endless litany of facts and then instantly forgetting them the day after the exam to make room for the next set. Any potential joy of learning is easily thwarted by the sheer volume of information flow. While I understand the importance of a strong foundation in science to eventually serve patients, those first few months of school made me feel like I was on a path devoid of any greater meaning or appreciation of what it means to be human.

But then came the clinical exam room. In the midst of these unrelenting facts and multiple-choice tests, we have a weekly, four-hour reprieve to learn the "art" of medicine in a class called "Doctoring." Doctoring, as a verb: how to be a doctor. In the clinical exam rooms, we work with standardized patients (actors trained to play the part of a patient under the careful eye of faculty mentors) to learn how to perform a physical exam, the hallmark of any visit to a doctor's office. Each visit begins with me knocking on that oak-paneled door, where I enter to meet an expectant standardized patient. Wearing my short white coat (the long ones will be earned when we are official doctors) and a stethoscope around my neck, I simultaneously return to the play-acting days of my three-year-old self and the beginning of a ritual I will move through for the rest of my career.

Learning to perform the physical exam is in diametric opposition to the lecture-style didactics of the rest of our education. We learn the nuances of inspection, palpation, and auscultation, memorizing a flow of maneuvers that we may not appreciate the full significance of (yet). My default modus operandi when faced with long lists of tasks, against my own wisdom, is a mental checklist to ensure all bases are covered.

This was me in early fall, learning to perform the cardiac physical exam and rattle off findings: inspecting the chest (no scarring, no devices, no abnormal pulsations), palpating the precordium (no heaves, no thrills), and auscultating—listening in the region of each heart valve for S1 and S2 (lub and dub). I listened, heard it, and promptly took off the stethoscope to declare that the standardized patient did, indeed, have a heartbeat.

I'm glad that Dr. H., my faculty leader, did not let me get away with that.

"Good, you heard it! And what did you hear?"

I knew I was listening for S1 and S2, the quintessential lub-dub, and I had heard this, so I said so. I was not expecting his follow-up to that, though:

"And what did it sound like?"

What *does* a heartbeat sound like? Our lecturers for the sequence had carefully discussed the slight variations of blips on an EKG—the pathologic significance of a Tennessee versus a Kentucky gallop in a heart's rhythm—and yet I did not have the language to honor what this standardized patient's run-of-the-mill lub-dub heartbeat sounded like.

Dr. H. offered some handy advice that afternoon. He said that when we auscultate the heart, we are not just listening for the *presence* of a heartbeat—every living patient is going to have that. We are listening for the *quality* of the beat. The nature of the rhythm, the space between the beats.

I took another try, placing the diaphragm of my stethoscope on the space between the first and second ribs, just to the right of the sternum. I closed my eyes, allowing time to move with the metronome of my patient's heart. I waited until I could hear the subtler tenor of the heartbeat below the more predominant tide of the breath. And in that moment, I heard so much more than just an S1 and S2. I was listening to the secrets of the engine that brought life to this standardized patient's body. Here, I was privy to the core of this person's physical self. While the write-up on this person's heart rhythm would merely state, "Normal heart sounds," in an essential, human way, this was a heartbeat unlike any other.

My first year is now drawing to a close. I still experience occasional weeks where I wonder whether I am on a career path that aligns with my beliefs about health and healing. But there are a lot more weeks where I can feel the ways in which my perspective fits into the evolving paradigm of modern medicine. What I have come to appreciate now, even in the lecture topics that seem far removed from the human aspect of medicine, is the intrinsic awe that drives this field forward. Whether it is in the tangible expression of the negative pressure that creates space for the symmetric breath I felt on my first full, standardized patient exam, or in the exact molecular mechanism that makes fatty acid metabolism possible, our work here is grounded in the fascination with life itself. It is an ongoing process, but one of upward personal and professional growth, and for that, I am thankful.

The Widowmaker

Jack Buchanan

If modern medicine were a patient, his chief concern would be chest pain. And he wouldn't be just any man, but the real stoic kind, like the hyper-stereotyped heroes you see in movies about Spartan warriors and Roman gladiators. But he'd also be like the traditional, hardworking types you know in real life, who can't be bothered much with eating salads or self-reflection (because that's just not what men do) and end up middle-aged with cardiovascular disease—and chest pain.

I made two big life decisions 11 years ago, near my halfway mark in college. First, I wanted nothing to do with medicine, for good. And second, I wanted everything to do with the French Alps, for at least a year. So I bracketed my human biology major, packed my snowboard, and traded the sunny shores of San Diego for the jutting snowcaps of Grenoble, France. On the way to the airport, I remember trying to explain to my father that medicine probably wasn't for me. I liked biology, to be sure, but my love for the outdoors and desire to protect it was pulling me in the direction of ecology and environmental studies.

My father was a geologist by training and a quintessential outdoorsman, so I could detect a layer of empathy behind the perfunctory paternalism:

"What do you plan to actually *do* with that kind of degree?" (in other words, "How will you make money?").

I didn't have an answer to his question, and frankly I didn't care. I was minutes away from embarking on what was about to be the greatest adventure of my life. I sensed the question was mostly rhetorical, anyway. Deep down I knew my father would support me in whatever I decided to do, so long as I fully applied myself.

At the time, there were precisely two things I was ready to fully apply myself to: snowboarding and Francophilia. That year abroad— the first time I'd set foot outside of North America—would be a true coming-of-age. At 19 years old, I found my own place to live; navigated French bureaucracy to obtain housing assistance; resolved a heated misunderstanding with a new roommate; and completed coursework in ecology, psychology, and political science—all in a foreign language. I learned much of what I now know about cooking through pure imitation and launched a sweeping sortie into the hinterlands of French cheese (it's true when they say there's a new kind for every day of the year). I celebrated Carnival in Cologne as a gypsy, ate mushrooms in Vondelpark, and carved bluebird powder on top of Mont Blanc. But none of these experiences was as transformative as a single phone call at the end of my year abroad.

Psychologists say memory formation is greatly enhanced during moments of peak distress. I will certainly never forget the moment I received the news. I was at my desk in my bedroom, cramming for my second-to-last final exam, on the social psychology of motivation. I had only a couple more hours before the test and a lot left to review. It was around 9 a.m., and I had just poured a quick bowl of cereal (the French equivalent of Kellogg's Special K Red Berries) so I wouldn't have to test on an empty stomach. A few bites in, my cell phone rang. I wouldn't have picked up had it not been an American number. From my mother's subdued tone, I knew immediately bad news loomed. Her cadence was fraught with hesitation, as if she herself had become confused about the reason for her call. Filled with curiosity and dread, I grew impatient.

"Please just tell me, Mom. Whatever it is."

She paused and drew a breath. At the age of 69, while playing handball, my father had suffered a massive heart attack leading to cardiac arrest and immediate death. At first, the words did not compute: how could he just be gone, in an instant? An overwhelming sense of loss started to bear down on my chest like a steel plate, padded with neither warning nor goodbye. My heart raced. My breath grew strained and shallow. Tears streamed until my eyes matched the red berry mush staring back at me from the bottom of the cereal bowl. Flashing memories of my father, already distant in space, tore open a gap in time. For the first time, eternity punctuated my finite existence rather than the other way around. Shock gradually gave way to the sting of cognitive acceptance, but physically internalizing that acceptance would take some time. For minutes after hanging up with my mother, the news fully sunken in, my whole body shook.

Autopsy would reveal myocardial infarction secondary to thrombus of the proximal left anterior descending (LAD) coronary artery. The LAD is the largest and most critical of the coronary arteries, as it supplies blood to the heart's most muscular chamber, the left ventricle. The left ventricle, in turn, bears the phenomenal burden of delivering oxygen to virtually every cell in the body, including its own. I would later learn that doctors have nicknamed the LAD the "widowmaker" because of the high mortality rate associated with heart attacks caused by its failure.[1] So my father's LAD had lived up to its medical moniker: its failure killed him, leaving my mother without her life partner. If an LAD heart attack is common enough to have its own nickname, the fact that my family was only now learning of its importance, and in such callous terms, seemed to add insult to injury.

---

1   If someone is fortunate enough to make it to the hospital alive following occlusion of the widowmaker, their EKG (which graphs the electrical conduction patterns of the heart) will show a characteristic shape that physicians refer to as the "tombstone" pattern. Cute, right?

I wondered about the reactions of other families for whom a similar tragedy had realized this preordained fate.[2]

In retrospect, my father's death marked the beginning of my decade-long arc back to medicine. I now see the subsequent journey as a process of reconciling my own identity with my father's legacy. Our relationship had been complicated—he embodied some values I proudly shared, but others I did not. As a child, I was a typical "mama's boy," and he and my brother took much delight in teasing me for it. Perhaps I bonded better with my mother because I take after her much more than I do my father, who in many ways was her polar opposite. Where my mother is thoughtful, meticulous, and analytic, my father was swift, brash, and decisive. Where she appreciates complexity and values dialogue, he tended to see the world in black and white, imploring me to always "Tell it like it is" and "Do it the right way" (with the clear implication that there is, in fact, just one way). Where she tended to lead from the heart, he endorsed a sort of detached rationality and ridiculed those who he saw as its direct adversaries: "do-gooder" types who use "touchy-feely" rhetoric to argue right versus wrong.

Language matters. Words serve as portals into the inner worlds of their speakers, reflecting deep-seated biases in the perspectives of whole cultures as well as single individuals. Just as my father's language betrayed his underlying hostility toward softer ways of coming to know one's world and the proper relations within it, the widowmaker reveals an ontological bias in modern medicine: that in some important sense, states of disease are more real (and therefore more important) than states of health. As a medical student, I learn to appreciate the body and its parts—even the most crucial, life-sustaining ones—most for how they fail. In this way, we inadvertently gain a sort of irreverent reverence for dysfunction. And as the

2   I also wonder how the term is received by families of individuals affected by a "widowmaker" heart attack who aren't male, married, and/or straight.

de facto gatekeepers of medical terminology, physicians encode this bias into vernacular legacies that diffuse throughout the healthcare ecosystem and reproduce themselves across time.

Medicine's fixation on dysfunction neither arose nor persists in a vacuum; it grows in tandem with a culture of provider stoicism that can give way to subtle self-effacement. Put differently, the more complicit providers become with the notion that health only becomes relevant in its overt absence, the more self-care is viewed as superfluous, and vice versa. Few would disagree that the needs of sick patients take precedence over those of their ostensibly well providers, but rarely are the limits of this truism explored. At what extreme does provider suffering command the same level of compassionate care as that of patients? The answer cannot be the point at which hardship interferes with patient care, because by then it's too late—for both patient and provider. The insight required to preempt such a situation depends on the very same capacity that the dysfunction bias calls into question—namely, an ability to recognize the insidiousness of merely less-than-well states. Perhaps these dynamics driving the valorization of self-sacrifice can help explain why physician burnout—a condition characterized by a loss of enthusiasm for work, feelings of cynicism, and a low sense of personal accomplishment—has become as pervasive as it is taboo. As simultaneous recipient and supplier of the heart's blood, the LAD artery has a simple lesson to teach us in this regard: *that one must be nourished in order to nourish others.* We must no longer think of wellness as a luxury good in a zero-sum marketplace, but instead as an essential and renewable resource whose benefits extend far beyond the individual.

The dysfunction bias also affects patient care directly. It is no secret that modern allopathic medicine in the U.S. spends far more time, energy, and resources on curative care than it does on prevention; this is by design. Existing efforts to shift the balance toward lower-tech but higher-value care, where value is measured not just in dollar savings but in human welfare, need to both deepen and broaden until they soak the very fabric of medical culture and reach beyond the walls of the clinic. Thinking back to the years preceding my father's death, I wonder if the outcome would have been different had his primary care physician, even in the absence of symptoms, engaged him in more dialogue around the importance of diet and preventive screenings. Imagining more broadly, what if the next generation of physicians could establish ourselves in the minds of our patients not only as technicians of chest pain, but also as trusted partners, role models, and leaders in a shared quest for longevity and well-being?

I ultimately chose to return, full circle, to medicine because I saw the seeds of such a shift already being sown. I saw an opportunity to integrate the values of empathy, dialogue, and self-compassion that I inherited from my mother, with the pointed rationality, driving work ethic, and stoic altruism that I admired in my father. Here at the University of Michigan where I attend medical school, I see an active recalibration of medicine underway—a rebalancing of rationalism with compassion, knowing with feeling, doing with being, talking with listening, and leading with collaborating. The curriculum provides us with various opportunities to engage with our own medical education in ways that will hopefully allow us to shift the culture of medicine through leadership and example.

After a turbulent transition to the first year of medical school, I was finally beginning to find more solid footing by the time I returned home for Thanksgiving break. This year it was only Mom and me, celebrating Thanksgiving in conjunction with her 72nd birthday. I had just completed my cardiology sequence, and I asked her if I could take a look at Dad's autopsy report. Now with a much more discerning eye than when I first saw it nine years ago, I found a strange solace as I took in the impersonalized jargon of the report: "thrombus of left hand and descending coronary artery due to calcific coronary artery atherosclerosis." In that moment, reading the post-mortem condition of my father's body, I felt at peace. As cold and mechanical as the language of the report was, there was something beautiful about the simple, factual sequence of physiologic events that had led to my father's death—something that afforded me a sense of closure I hadn't been able to secure before.

At the time of writing, the 10th anniversary of my father's death is approaching. As my personal journey of reconciliation draws toward a close, I begin to reflect on the steps that my peers and I, as the next generation of physicians, can take to positively shape the future of medicine. It is incumbent on us to ensure that reverence, humility, and stewardship for the human body are thoroughly reflected in the formal institutions of medicine as well as in their linguistic encodements. For the former, we must affirm the importance of self-care and the value of prevention throughout medical education, training, and practice. For the latter, we must abandon loaded terms such as widowmaker, which perpetuate outmoded paradigms and betray a callous disconnect from patients' lived experiences. Like my meat-and-potatoes father before his heart attack, the patient who presents with chest pain at the beginning of this story is in need of significant lifestyle changes. But unlike my father, this patient need not worry about survival per se, so much as quality of life. For while the enterprise of medicine is likely to persist as long as humans do, neither the timelessness of its science nor the transcendence of its art will ever translate into immunity from worldly dysfunction. The first step in any self-betterment is a good honest look in the mirror.

A Twinge of Discomfort

Nithya Vijayakumar

Intravenous Line Workshop. The nurse gives us instructions. Tighten band on upper arm. Feel for strong veins, like rope under skin. Clean field with alcohol swab. Insert needle along vein. Push cannula in; retract needle. Pull syringe back. Watch blood rush through tubing and swirl with sterile saline. Push saline in.

In the basement of our medical school, surrounded by cement walls and black lab benches, I repeat these steps under my breath quietly. My fingers model the movements, and my partner and I stare at each other in a silent test of wills. As I worry that my inexperience will cause the insertion to go terribly wrong, my mouth blurts out, "You can go first." With nervous laughter, she begins and executes perfectly. The insertion is (almost) painless, which eases my fear. I step forward.

Focused on the contraption in front of me, I proceed with an eye on my partner's face for signs of discomfort. The insertion goes smoothly. I'm relieved once it's over, surprised by my own success. We take photos of our handiwork. Barely three months into medical school, I am thankful she entrusted me with her vein and hopeful the next time will be less daunting. Looking around the room, I don't know if other students feel similarly.

I like to imagine this basement as a renovated fight club—fluorescent lights, no windows, and 20 pairs of first-year medical students inserting needles into each other's arms. There would be many more hours studying in this basement over the coming year.

One floor above the basement, old fixtures shine fluorescent light over my classmates on our first day of anatomy. I'd been excited about this for weeks—older physicians never failed to mention how gross anatomy is a formative stepping stone into medicine, the first stripe on our belts toward becoming *doctors*. In a large laboratory that smells of preservation, we approach our cadavers and adjust the lab coats we are given. Some of these coats have stains or embroidered names of former physicians. Five students stand around the body of a deceased man, gazing in wonder and trepidation. We first appreciate the marks on his skin—the tattoo on his forearm and age spots around his neck—and the sparse strands of hair decorating his body. We look at his cause of death. When it comes time to cut, we hesitate. I rest one hand gently on our donor's back, holding the scalpel in the other.

I am not sure if I'm ready to unravel the intricate organization of his body, to learn intimate parts of his being that he shared with those he trusted. Though he had much to teach us, his most important stories about living would remain untold after his death. We would barely scratch the surface of his life. One student cuts in bravely, surprised at the toughness of skin after preservation. I join in making an incision, and like that, the human body becomes something to explore. The coming months reveal metastasized tumors, hernias, aortic aneurysms, benign kidney cysts, and the nuanced variation in vascular and neurologic organization from person to person. I would marvel at the thoracic cavity, eager to hold the muscular heart walls and trace vasculature with my fingertips. I would step back when we unraveled our cadaver's intestines because my own threatened to unravel inside of me. Our donor gave his body so we could learn from him even when he could no longer speak. As I leave anatomy lab, I let this privilege leave heavy footprints in my mind, hoping my acquaintance with his body will help me better understand and serve the bodies of my patients.

Perhaps these repeatedly uncomfortable experiences are a warm-up for a lifelong career in medicine that incessantly pushes us beyond our boundaries.

A few months later, we learn the male genitourinary and female pelvic exams with the aid of standardized patients, who are trained to teach us these sensitive exams. My partner and I walk into a simulated exam room where fluorescent lights cast blue shadows, and my perennially cold fingertips appear colorless. I wonder if the blood has left my hands the way half of me wants to leave the room. Our standardized patient greets us. I apologize for my freezing hands and wonder how well coldness transfers through gloves. After examining the external genitalia, we move on to the digital rectal exam. We discuss the exam, and I register his ordinary professionalism next to my unease. He has known me for 20 minutes, and yet he trusts me enough to curl into the fetal position facing away from me. I prepare the field and slide purple nitrile gloves over my hands. I take a deep breath. I watch his face as I imagine he braces himself. Facing away, he cannot see exactly what I am doing, and I hesitate at this vulnerability. A part of me seems to be observing from the vantage of the fluorescent lights above us—two students in short, white coats, who seem so small when faced with a trust that seems so large.

Our standardized patient provides instruction and feedback throughout, and I follow along. "Insert a gloved, well-lubricated index finger gently through the anus into the rectum. Palpate the prostate to assess for masses and consistency. Using a firm, slow motion, palpate all around the rectal walls, noting the texture." We had practiced earlier on a plastic model, but there are few ways to be fully prepared. We are told that prostate cancer may feel like a hard, woody nodule, but a healthy prostate feels like the tip of your nose. A mass in the rectum could suggest colorectal cancer. I am tempted to finish this invasive procedure quickly, worried about causing him discomfort. He encourages us to be thorough, to learn as much as possible for future patients. After we finish, we thank him many times for teaching us, trusting us, and offering to be vulnerable so that we may learn.

Leaving the exam simulation room, I walk home in crisp January air. As medical students, we spend a lot of time in windowless rooms under fluorescent lights. Perhaps it is the nature of this work, to keep secrets within walls when they are no longer kept within skin. Few are privy to the pathologies that take place underneath skin's surface, but our teachers, patients, donors, friends, and occasionally even passersby, share their stories and bodies with us. This is the responsibility I wrestle with—to be a body's healer, earning and upholding the trust of its owner. Perhaps as I learn more, I will become more confident and comfortable. Perhaps the trust our patients give us will begin to feel normal. However, I hope a twinge of discomfort will always remind me of the privilege I hold.

The Alarming Resistance of Medical Student Choices to Bayesian Analysis

Mason Shaner

On Sunday, April 30, I look up at the corner of my computer screen: 10:57 p.m. I need to make a decision. Seemingly seconds pass, and the computer displays 11:30 p.m. I have 30 minutes to make a choice. A choice that will, without doubt, open some doors and close others; I cannot possibly know which ones.

I glance at my neatly formatted list of variables once again, a document that seems to overly simplify this difficult task. Do I stay in San Diego, an area I have called home for nearly a decade, or do I pull up roots to go to Ann Arbor? These considerations include tuition, living costs, debt, family responsibilities, my allegiance to the inner-city high school students I taught before applying to medical school (and their families), estimated likelihood of being happy, the quality of the medical school program, and the list continues. Each variable is multiplied by a value factor with an underlying theory I'm not sure I quite fully grasp.

Index finger shaking, I select the University of Michigan. Submit. I fake a sigh of relief. I choose, for the first time, to leave Southern California.

For me, making big decisions always has been difficult. I am a pros-and-cons-list kind of person who likes to have a plethora of information in order to make a reasoned choice based on objective expectations. I am great to have around during brainstorming, planning, and development, and a pain in quick decision-making. This technique has served me well in teaching high school for two years at an inner-city school where a lack of preparation can cost you your relationship with students. I credit my training in biomedical engineering for helping me with decision-making and acknowledge my futile attempts to use Bayesian analysis, plagued by problems of over-fitting, to solve my personal dilemmas.

Bayesian analysis can be thought of as updating the likelihood of a hypothesis to be true as more information or evidence becomes available. For example, here is a hypothesis: "I will be happier going to Ann Arbor for medical school than staying in San Diego." The way I look at it, one can combine prior probabilities based on experience with current observations to make an informed decision about the likely answer to the question about how best to proceed.

Whew! What a relief. I stand up and stretch, my decision made. Now I think: I am lucky. It should be straightforward in medical school. Relax a bit. Fewer difficult choices. I have an adventure in front of me, and I'll rise to the occasion. I've already made the tough decision.

After our class's White Coat Ceremony, I felt even more firmly positioned on the path to becoming a physician, leaving the winding, tangled, and uncertain byway behind. I felt excited to be gaining knowledge that would help me to become the best physician I can be. I knew also that, at the University of Michigan, the pre-clinical curriculum is compressed, condensed, and squeezed into one year. Good, I thought. Less is more. Little did I think about the precious commodity time would become as a result and the odd impact this would have on my values and priorities. While time in the past always had been valuable, suddenly it became a scarcity, and never "free." How to spend it became a daily quandary.

My first decision was whether to attend lectures. I did at first, but my background in education meant I could not help but notice the difficulties some professors had with teaching—possessing a deep command of the material but perhaps lacking formal education in teaching technique. Other medical students offered that they streamed the material online or even pre-streamed content from last year. I began to question my decision; could I have learned this content better or faster if I had stayed home? I quickly realized there was enough to memorize that inefficient time management could impede good test performance and reduce opportunities for recreation, personal care, or fostering relationships.

Confident, I turned to a pros-and-cons list as my usual go-to approach: attending lecture allowed me to interact with classmates who I might otherwise not have seen, while staying home allowed me to view lecture content at a faster or slower pace to optimize my time. As my analysis proceeded in this mundane manner, I soon realized I lacked sufficient information to make this choice. The questions I considered included how proficient the lecturer might be, how reliable the streaming equipment would be on the given day, and the prioritizing of other responsibilities to which I needed to attend. Nagging at me in all of this remained one professor's passing comment and a plea for a socially responsible solution: if we as medical students wish for better and more interactive lectures and speakers, we should attend lectures to demonstrate to our speakers the lecture's importance to us. How, then, might my seemingly inconsequential decision to attend lecture affect others and future medical classes?

Just as I settled into an approach to the lecture schedule—deciding to attend the known, creative, or interesting talks and streaming the rest—we began anatomy. Students from the medical, dental, nursing, and physician assistant schools attend the Anatomical Donations Program Memorial Service, an event for the friends and families of those who have donated their bodies for student dissection. Perhaps the impending exams had forced a choice for many students, as I noticed most students left when the program ended rather than talking with attendees as instructed, even leaving the appealing free appetizers untouched.

As I considered whether to spend the precious time to mingle or to return to my studies, I looked around uncertainly, only to incidentally make eye contact with an elderly woman. She smiled toward me. Caught up in the moment, I walked over, my choice made. The families I spoke to seemed happy to talk about their loved ones and to learn about me. I felt glad I remained. When I later performed less well than I would have liked on that week's exam, I wondered: would I have been able to do better had I not stayed? Did it matter? Did I make a difference to that elderly woman?

I spend hours at the library every day, memorizing, studying, and reviewing with others to master the content. I work harder than I ever have in my life, still honing skills to use my time best. With each quiz and exam result, the question becomes: what choices did I make that week? When I was a high school teacher, my hard work translated quickly to success. Here, I see an uncertain and seemingly arbitrary benefit in test scores. While teaching, I spent months writing an entire high school medical chemistry curriculum and then implementing it in an under-resourced public charter school. Students told me they appreciated learning about real-life concepts and were excited to come to class—a feeling that carried me through the late nights, hard days, and difficult interactions with families and the administration. The pros and cons were not always easy to discern, but I rarely questioned my decisions. Now in medical school, I often feel ill-equipped to make decisions about spending my time productively and have had scant opportunity to reflect on those choices.

One of our lecturers pointed out that the decisions we make now will affect us over the next 50 years of our lives. Every week, we have lunch talks, during which a panel of physicians from a given specialty discuss why they chose the specialty and outline details about residency applications. Although I may be drawn to a number of these specialties, I understand also that some residencies are more competitive than others, and I should have started building my application for them, well, yesterday. The celebration I felt in finally getting into medical school seemed overshadowed by a new, potentially convoluted path, one that became less definite as my confidence in my methodical approach to decision-making waned. Third- and fourth-year medical students reassure me that during my second year, a specialty will quickly "pop out" to me, and the decision will be clear and unequivocal—no pros-and-cons list needed. I'm thinking this is like the hat in Harry Potter that directs the student. Really? Optimistically, I hope they are right.

I spoke to fellow medical students in my class about how ambiguity affects us. Some confessed that they questioned their decision to become physicians. One student considered leaving before completing half of our first year. Another student commented that this year has been easier in some ways than previous undergraduate years. However, for the majority, the confidence felt after the White Coat Ceremony had evaporated. In this atmosphere of uncertainty, medical students in classes ahead offered us, nonchalantly, that this first year is the easiest.

With time, I have abandoned pros-and-cons lists. I persevere based on a recipe of optimism, blind faith, and a return to the initial feeling that propelled me into medical school. My fellow medical students may find their own unique motivations. Sustaining me is my belief and hope that, at some future time, I will find a way to help underserved students, like those I once taught and still keep in touch with, desperately in need of improved health-care access and health-care literacy.

With this approach, I find myself reflecting on the decisions I have made and those I must make. Where will my medical career take me, and in which specialty? I feel lucky to have freedom to make such choices. That said, when a choice's foundations are unclear or its consequences dimly foreseeable, when time constraints create a dilemma between choosing what is quick and what is right, when an abundance of creative alternatives complicate a straightforward path, you may be in medical school.

Unabashedly Unprepared

Erika Steensma

I am standing in a chilly room filled with steel tables, dingy baskets of surgical equipment, and more dead people than I have ever seen in my life. The bitter taste of coffee is in my mouth, and my stomach turns—I am instantly regretting that second cup I had this morning before my first anatomy lab. My dissecting partner hands me the scalpel, and I slowly swivel to face the stiff man lying on the table in front of me. I swallow hard and hesitate, bracing myself for the first cut. At this moment, my normal flood of thoughts disintegrates and only one sentiment blares through my mind: I have no idea what I am doing.

As the first person in my family to attend medical school, I was naturally anxious about all that the experience would entail. Yet in the months prior to the start of classes, anatomy was the subject that most terrified me. I had nightmares of dimly lit labs filled with cadavers and décor better fit for a medieval-period horror movie than a modern medical school. Therefore, with trepidation I entered the anatomy lab for the first time. The experience was, at the same time, everything and nothing like I expected.

The large, drafty room had stark white walls and was illuminated with bright fluorescent lights, the kind that ensure no one standing under them looks their best. I felt a small thrill when I noticed the rows of white laboratory coats hanging along the side walls, one of which would soon become mine; although I had no idea what I was doing, at least I would look like a professional while doing it. Being the germophobe that I am, I was also relieved to see multiple hand-washing stations throughout the room. However, these vague reassurances could not overpower the horror I experienced when I glanced at a nearby bookcase and found myself staring at rows of severed human limbs that had been immaculately preserved for teaching purposes. And then, of course, there was the matter of the donor bodies.

When I reached my dissection table, I initially attributed the chill that ran through my body as a reaction to the stiff, sheet-covered figure lying on the table in front of me. However, a glance upward soon revealed the true cause: I was standing directly beneath a ceiling ventilator that was pumping cold air across the back of my neck. Although the source of my chill had been identified, the source of my unease was still lying in front of me. There is something fundamentally disturbing about standing before the deceased body of a fellow human being and realizing you will soon be cutting away all of their muscles and organs in an attempt to understand their basic anatomy.

At the University of Michigan Medical School, the anatomists try their hardest to normalize the anatomy experience and guide students through the process. Our first day did not involve any scalpels or scissors; rather, we had a 30-minute session to meet the faculty, the teaching assistants (second-year medical students who had completed this course the previous year), and our donors. The anatomy program is made possible by the incredible sacrifice of men and women who willingly donate their deceased bodies to further the education of medical students. Following the donors' deaths, their bodies are prepared for dissection and assigned to eight-person groups of medical students. These groups then split into teams of four that alternate performing the dissections.

That first day, however, none of us could consider lifting a scalpel to the man lying before us. It was with clear discomfort that we tried to find the proper mindset for the dissection that would be occurring in the coming weeks. Should we consider our donor as a biological specimen and nothing more? Although this would make dissection easier, it seemed disrespectful toward a man who had, literally, given his entire body to better the education of students he would never meet. Yet viewing him as a fellow human being was equally disturbing; the thought of slicing a human into pieces is horrifying. We stood silently in front of our donor for 20 minutes, no one certain of what to say or think, and somberly left at the end of the session. It was in these moments that I came to the full realization that there are some aspects of medical school for which a person simply cannot be prepared.

On the morning of my first dissection, I showed up to school wearing my favorite bright pink scrubs, a memento from the nursing home I worked at in my life prior to medical school. I wanted my outfit to show a level of cheeriness I was not feeling inside. I was terrified for what I was about to do; our lab manual contained instructions such as "skin the neck to locate the sternocleidomastoid muscle"—words that left me lightheaded and nauseous. While most of that first session is a blur in my mind, I still remember that underlying sensation of malaise as the dissection began. One of my group members offered me the scalpel, asking if I would like to make the first cut. It was a gesture that I quickly declined; I was in no way willing to do this. He shrugged and immediately dove into the dissection with a vigor that both impressed and slightly repulsed me.

While I had mentally steeled myself to face the sights of dissection, I was not prepared for the accompanying noises and scents. Within moments, the air was filled with the stiff stench of preservatives, which seemed to permeate through my clothes and hair. After a series of cuts and several minutes of aggressive tugging, our group managed to finally yank the neck skin from the sternocleidomastoid muscle. As the skin reluctantly tore free, it was accompanied by a loud, wet, slurping noise. The teaching assistant smiled at us as she passed.

"Don't you just love that sound!" she exclaimed, "I just find it so satisfying."

I remained silent, focusing all my attention on keeping my sloshing breakfast within my stomach and taking a quick inventory of nearby trashcans, just in case I would need to make a dash for one. No, satisfying was not the word I would have used to describe that moment.

Frustrated by my fear and fueled by a desire to prove I was capable of completing the requirements of medical school, I forced myself to take a more active role in the dissection. I requested the scalpel and, with a quaking hand, made a very unsteady slice through the skin on the donor's back. I was surprised at how smoothly the skin separated beneath the blade, and even more amazed at how natural it felt to be using a scalpel. "I *can* do this," I thought, a realization driven more by shock than confidence. I, furthermore, learned the value of distraction in adapting to anatomy. By diverting all my attention to differentiating the phrenic nerve from the vagus nerve, and intercostal arteries from intercostal veins, I was able to conveniently forget about the more disturbing aspects of the dissection. I'm not sure when the transition occurred, but two hours into the lab, I slowly came to the realization that I no longer was horrified by everything. As it turns out, the most bizarre aspect of anatomy lab, for me, was how swiftly it stopped being bizarre and became natural.

I cannot explain how it happens, but at some point in the dissection process, the mind adapts to its gruesome nature. This process is different for everyone; some were able to dive right in, whereas others took days and weeks to adjust to the experience. And while I still do not particularly enjoy performing anatomy dissections, I have gained an appreciation for all that I learn while doing them. I have skinned my donor's back and marveled at the size of the muscles that lay beneath the surface. I have bemoaned the intricacy of his nerves while trying to separate them from adjacent structures, at the same time appreciating just how complex and incredible the human nervous system is. I have held his heart in my hand, wondering at the countless beats it once produced, sustaining a man who touched others while living and who is shaping me, even after his death. I have found that the key to accepting anatomy lab is not to choose whether to view my donor as a biological specimen or as a human, but to view him as both at the same time. Somehow, relating the dissection I am doing to the man who once lived and to my patients who I will one day treat allows me to justify my work.

I last stepped foot in the anatomy lab about two months ago for our class' final practical exam. These tests entail walking from table to table and identifying structures that have been fastidiously isolated and labeled by the anatomy faculty. Each student has 75 seconds to make the identification, after which a timer buzzes and everyone switches to the next station, ready or not. With the pressure of both a stringent time limit and an exam that could test almost any muscle, bone, or nerve in the body, I was understandably anxious as I circled through the laboratory. My mind was racing, trying to keep track of how many structures I had recognized or guessed on, and my heart was pounding; whether this was from adrenaline or too much coffee was unclear to me. I stepped in front of my next station, praying for an easy identification. As I glanced down at the pin sticking into the palm of a body's hand, I felt a slow smile creep across my face. I knew that hand, and by proxy, the thick muscle that the pin was plunging through. I was looking at the hand of my donor.

A sense of calm and peace came over me; I was looking at a familiar body, an almost friend. For the remaining 65 seconds, my eyes traced through his arms, his chest cavity, his neck, silently identifying the life-sustaining nerves and vessels that, one year ago, I didn't even know existed. The buzzer rang, and I felt an unexpected reluctance to leave his side for the last time ever. But as I left, I glanced back and sent a mental message to him, as if he could read my thoughts and understand my sentiment.

"Thank you," I told him silently. "Thank you for everything."

My Night Alone in the Anatomy Lab

Apoorv Dhir

One of the most anticipated experiences of the first year of medical school is anatomy lab. For most students, it is their first time observing a dead body and, to most, the experience is shocking. Spending time with—let alone dissecting—deceased human beings is anything but normal, yet we quickly grow accustomed to this macabre rite of passage, becoming more afraid of poor grades than we are of the dead.

Like many others, this was how my relationship with the cadavers began. I was truly terrified on my first day, sweating through my scrubs, worried that, after years of pushing through prerequisites, my fear of the dead would be what weeded me out on the long road to becoming a doctor. But, no! I didn't trudge through Physics 235 to attend only the first few days of medical school; I was committed for the long haul. So, I fought my fear of the dead as I had fought my fear of magnetic fields. Soon, I was cutting right alongside my classmates, more focused on finding the insertion points of *pectoralis major* than on contemplating the lost life lying on the other side of my latex gloves.

In the days leading up to our first anatomy practical, many people in our class were taking advantage of the anatomy lab as a study tool. As detailed as our textbooks are, there is no better way to identify structures on a human body than by studying them on an actual cadaver. So, I arranged to meet one of my friends in the anatomy lab the night before our practical.

I walked into the lab just after 11 p.m., the ominously late time at which we had agreed to meet. As I entered, I found a group of students finishing up their review and getting ready to leave—my friend among them. Through some miscommunication, he had come an hour before and decided to go on without me. I was left alone; no one else was willing to stay in the lab so late to study with me.

In this moment, I had two choices: leave now and wing it for my first anatomy practical or stay alone in a cold, dimly lit lab surrounded by dead bodies. I felt like I was walking into the first scene of a B-list horror film, but I knew what I had to do. I had come to medical school to absorb as much information as possible, and I would have felt silly turning down an opportunity to learn.

I set down my backpack by the coat hangers and slipped on a pair of gloves as the last of my classmates trickled out of the chilly lab. I focused my study on the skeletons at the front of the lab, finding comfort in their relative familiarity and normalcy. I mean, looking at real human bones is easy when you convince yourself you are just looking at insanely realistic Halloween decorations.

After studying the same bone for ten long minutes, I finally found the courage to make my way over to the body bag. As I prepared myself, I swore I could hear shuffling in the next room over. I perked up, first in pure joy of another living human by my side, and then in fear of the unearthly. Of course, the sounds were likely my mind's last defense against the inevitable. I lifted the sheet from the donor before me and began to study the skin, fat, and superficial muscles of his back.

As I busied myself in studying the donor's anatomy, I let my fear slip away. I sank into the fascinating architecture of the human body and got lost in its design. I examined the depths of all the different layers of tissue and marveled at the vertebral column, anxious to discover the precious spinal cord beneath. I followed muscles from origin to insertion, trying to engrain in my mind the orientation of their fibers. I felt for the different textures, contrasting the rigidity of bone to the meat of muscle to the pliability of fat. As the concept of my solitude resurfaced in my mind, I wrapped up my studying within 15 minutes and decided to get out of the lab.

I covered my donor, removed my gloves, and washed my hands, getting ready to leave. After I dried my hands, I took a moment to look around at all the tables. I reflected on how each table held the remains of a generous donor, posthumously gifting knowledge to dozens of curious medical students. In that moment of silence, the lab felt oddly serene.

In the lab by myself, surrounded by cadavers, I was alone. Scientifically speaking, there was no other living being in the same space as me. That was a fact. But I did not feel alone. The donors in the lab were not alive, but they were still human. When I was in the lab, I never felt as if I was studying *something*; I was always studying *someone*.

So far, in my early stages of medical training, I am learning that the art of medicine is a delicate balance between hard science and humanity. We bury our noses in books filled with long words describing every single way the human body can falter. Then, we carry this deep knowledge to everyday encounters with real people who cannot possibly be reduced to a section in a chapter of a textbook.

As I was studying that night, alone in the lab, I was able to dive into the science of anatomy and forget for a brief moment the truly terrifying nature of what I was doing. But ultimately, it is not that simple. Each donor has a life story I will never learn, but I will always appreciate. When I study my donor's stomach, I think of all the family dinners that may have passed through. When I look at a donor's hands, I think of the loved ones that donor may have held. At the end of the day, it motivates me to understand the science and anatomy of these past lives, so I can apply them to help those who are still living. It's a gift I truly appreciate and will never forget.

I grabbed my coat and bag and decided it was time to leave. I could finish whatever introspection I had begun outside the lab, but it was time to get back into the land of the living. Just as I was leaving and turning into another hall, I ran into another classmate.

Nervously, he asked, "Hey, I haven't had a chance to study in the lab yet, and I don't think there's anyone in there…will you go in with me?"

"Sure," I said, "Why not?"

A Poster Presentation

Anonymous

Poster presentations go something like this: posters full of figures and diagrams and blocks of text are lined up in neat rows. Presenters stand by, ready to explain their research. Presentation-goers mill around, moving slowly, reading titles, listening to explanations, sampling as if at an hors d'oeuvre party. In the scientific world, this is the formalized custom for bringing the community together to exchange viewpoints, discuss the newest innovations, and disseminate ideas. Medical students practice this too: first attending presentations to learn how research is discussed and, later, advancing to become presenters themselves.

The very first time I went to a medical school poster presentation, the first poster I stepped in front of had a title that went something like, "Exposure to Drunk Driving and Risk of Domestic Violence." The research was investigating whether children who have been in cars with drunk drivers are more likely to experience domestic violence. The presenter started explaining to me the hypothesis, the methods, and the conclusions he had reached. But I heard none of it, because my mind was racing back to the time when I was 15 and sitting in the back of my family's SUV.

The night had seemed so unremarkable up until the moment our car slowed to meet the police car. An officer stepped up to the driver's side window, and I watched as my father opened the door and left. I looked on as the blue-and-red police lights flashed all around.

I remember imagining my father trying to walk down a line in a parking lot, although the police officers had hidden that from my view. I curled up in the backseat and waited expectantly for my father to come back, certain this would be a short inconvenience. But hours stretched on, and my father never did come back. Instead, he was arrested and taken to jail. The car was impounded, and a neighbor came to take me home. There was a line on the poster explaining what drunk driving exposure meant, but I already knew.

Other memories flooded in: I remembered the days when the beer came out of the fridge in the afternoon, and by nighttime, my dad was frighteningly unpredictable. The morning when my brother showed me his stiff, swollen, broken fingers from the night before, and I held his small hands in mine and looked into his worried face, not knowing what to do. I remembered watching my dad push my mom, pinning her down to shout at her, and my mother, scared, telling me not to be scared, everything would be all right. And the handful of times when my dad was angry, so angry, I would leave the house and aimlessly wander the neighborhood for a few hours until I felt the storm had passed.

The presenter was still telling me about his research, but his words all slipped away from me. I stood there, mind rushing through a long reel of memories, trying my best to give the impression I was listening until the presenter seemed to have made his way through all of his talking points. He paused and looked at me, and I looked back. If words exist to sum up what I was feeling at that moment, I couldn't come up with them. I wanted to tell him that I knew exactly what he was talking about, that he didn't need to define or clarify his terms to me. And I wanted to explain how shocking it was to have found myself in front of a poster that spoke to me so vividly. It was as if I had picked up a textbook and found inside it a description of my childhood home. I wanted to ask about how he had chosen that topic of research or ask if he had ever experienced or imagined experiencing any of the things he was researching. I wanted to thank him for spending his entire summer illuminating a piece of this phenomenon that had wreaked so much havoc on my childhood. I wanted to say all of this, but I could think of no way to say it professionally. So I settled on a woefully inadequate, "I'd like to do research like this someday," and left.

Domestic violence and alcoholism exist at an awkward intersection—one the medical field is aware of but dark family secrets and social convention make it difficult to acknowledge. Domestic violence is something medical students do learn about—doctors are responsible for reporting possible abuse or violence in the home when clinical suspicion suggests it. And yet, so few are comfortable talking about domestic violence. In my training, I have met medical students and physicians alike who shy away from conversations about domestic violence with their patients in all but the most extreme cases. Perhaps some of that hesitation is because our society has not yet found a "cure" for it; there is precious little known about how to prevent domestic violence from happening. What's more, it's often hard to know how to stop domestic violence once it starts or how to help a victim who relies on an abuser for financial support, a home, a social network, or as a parenting partner. As a rule, there are no easy solutions, and that makes it tough to even start conversations about domestic violence.

Even fewer medical professionals are willing to talk about personal experiences with domestic violence. Domestic violence is simply not a polite topic of conversation, and its survivors don't often inspire awe for having survived it. In fact, survivors (including myself) can count on being questioned about whether their abuse really happened, why they put up with abuse for so long, why they didn't leave their abuser, or why they didn't just do *something* differently. All that doubt creates social inertia that can make it excruciatingly difficult to talk about domestic violence to patients, to friends, or to colleagues. I remember this every time I am asked to learn about domestic violence in a formal classroom setting, and I am faced with the choice of how to respond.

On the one hand, choosing to explain my story allows me to humanize domestic violence to my peers. For many people, domestic violence is usually imagined as something profoundly distant from normal, everyday lives. That perceived distance, the unwillingness to believe it could happen to a friend or an acquaintance, allows domestic violence to go unrecognized even in close proximity. I learned, growing up, how hard it was for my family's friends and neighbors to see domestic violence in my middle-class family and to recognize my successful physician father as an abusive alcoholic. It's my hope that if I am able to speak about my childhood experiences in the right ways, then I will broaden people's perspectives of what domestic violence is. And I hope those I speak to about it will be better equipped to see domestic violence in all of its non-stereotypical forms.

On the other hand, choosing to explain also means reliving my most private memories in front of friends and colleagues. It means spending months and years wondering what my classmates really think of me and my family and my stories. It means seeing the unspoken questions in friends' eyes and wondering how I can answer them. It means singling myself out as other, different. Sometimes, making the choice to speak out feels impossibly difficult.

I keep wondering if there will be a time when having conversations about what went on in my house during my childhood will feel easy. A time when I won't feel powerless under the force of my own memories. A time when I won't alienate anyone with my stories or find myself challenged by listeners who think my childhood "wasn't really all that bad." Among all my career goals as a physician, this is my dearest: that I may be able to have conversations about domestic violence that will promote better health for all survivors.

Until then, I live in the in-between, in the liminal space between my professional life and my personal life, between directing conversations about domestic violence and being the subject of them, between the privilege of my life as a medical student and the hardships of surviving long enough to make it here. I live with the quiet revelations of poster presentations and with the perpetual decision of whether to keep or tell my secrets.

The Parts of a Body

Hanna Saltzman

I.

Mrs. K. sat in a chair in the corner of the sterile cystic fibrosis room, arms and legs crossed, eyes cast downward, examining her fingernails. The dietician questioned her, and I sat nearby observing the interaction as part of my Initial Clinical Experience, in which first-year medical students shadow different members of the healthcare team. We'd been warned, the dietician and I, about this "crazy patient in room 13," by the pulmonologist who had just seen her. "Crazy" because she thought alternative medicine could fix her problems and was trying all sorts of "bogus" therapies. He had wished us luck in a tone halfway between frustrated and bewildered, moving on to his next patient.

In the room, I caught glimpses of Mrs. K.'s life through the lens of food: she's trying to eat more yogurt and chicken, fewer chips and Snickers bars, because she's upset about the weight she's gaining with menopause. Cooking has been a struggle because infections have trapped her in the house for the past several months. Michigan winters can be hard for patients with cystic fibrosis, and Mrs. K. is about to head off to California for a few months of sun and fresh fruit. The dietician commented on how much she admired Mrs. K.'s resilience for dealing with menopause and cystic fibrosis at the same time. Mrs. K.'s eyes moved from her fingernails to our faces.

"See, you get it, don't you?" she said softly. "He didn't."

"Who didn't?"

"That doctor! He wouldn't even talk to me…"

"What do you mean?"

"He wouldn't…. he wouldn't even let me say the word menopause… he thinks I'm just…" Mrs. K. leaned forward with flashing eyes, voice rising. "I'm not just lungs! I'm a whole human! A whole goddamn human! And you know what? When I gain weight in menopause I gain it right *here*." (She gestured frantically over her chest.) "Which means it's sitting right on top of my lungs, which makes it hard to breathe, which means it *is* connected to my cystic fibrosis, but he won't talk about it. He thinks I'm crazy. He literally rolled his eyes at me as if I wouldn't notice…I'm not a goddamn walking pair of lungs!"

In that moment, Mrs. K. took one of my biggest apprehensions about the process of medical school—learning through an educational schema that often views people as body parts rather than integrated humans, and thus unintentionally starting to view people that way myself—and plucked it out of my mind, where it had been growing for months. The way we learn medicine in our pre-clinical curriculum is primarily through short stints of delving deeply into one body part at a time: two weeks on the lungs, two weeks on the kidneys, three on the heart. Perhaps this type of conceptual disarticulation of bodies is necessary to master the colossal amount of information needed to become an excellent physician. But as a first-year student, this learning method already has started to transform how I see bodies, from whole to parts, and I have started to wonder to what extent I will be able to re-learn how to see people as whole again.

After clinic, I took my lungs to a yoga class. "Breathe through your entire lung space, bottom and top, back and sides," the teacher's voice floated across the room as I folded myself into child's pose. "Our breath is where it all begins, where it all ends. We are our breath."

An image cut through my mind: lungs attached to a bare skeleton, traipsing down the street—a walking pair of lungs. Focusing on my lungs at the yoga teacher's direction, I couldn't help thinking about the lungs of the patients I had seen in this first year of medical school. My patients' specific lung diseases entered my mind first (cystic fibrosis, emphysema), and then details of their lives trickled in second (the joy of my patient with cystic fibrosis who finally got pregnant, the pride of my patient with emphysema when speaking about her farm). Disease first, person second. That's how these humans entered my mind. This way of thinking has become my new reality, and its permanence is my fear.

II.

When the man who would become my anatomy donor (cadaver) died, per his wishes, his body entered through the back entrance of our anatomy lab. He was pumped full of preserving fluids, stapled with an ear-tag of "5-2," and accompanied by a note listing his age and what diseases he had died with: colon cancer and dementia, among other illnesses. His body was then stuck under a white sheet for first-year medical student anatomy group #5-2 to claim with our scalpels and excitement and anxieties. Time to meet our "first patient," we're told. Patient #5-2.

Two groups of students were assigned to each donor, alternating dissection days. After dissecting, each group presented their work to the other group. As I was assigned to the second group, I walked into the lab at the end of the first dissection for the presentation. In front of me was a ritual that seemed simultaneously sacred and profane, defying my ability to categorize it. Students in brightly colored scrubs cast aside white sheets and pored over the gray bodies of their "first patients." Holding scalpels and scissors, they followed the lab manual's instructions on skinning: piling slabs of skin into a bucket to be preserved for now and ultimately cremated. It's necessary, of course, for dissectors to remove the skin of the body in order to then explore the organs and vessels beneath it, to learn the magic that had enabled this human to live. But watching the skinning repulsed me.

The only other time I'd felt remotely similar was the day in college I volunteered to help process slaughtered chickens as part of an anthropology research project on small-scale farming. As I wasn't quite comfortable participating in the slaughter itself but still wanted to be involved, the farmer assigned me the post-slaughter task of chopping off the chickens' feet and throwing them into a bucket. After a few dozen chickens, a cold nausea came on, to the point that I couldn't stand up and had to leave, embarrassed by my inadequacy. For days afterwards, I continued to smell blood on my jacket and hands no matter how often I washed them. In that first medical school anatomy lab, I felt the same cold nausea and, afterwards, the same urgent need to wash, wash, wash myself to no avail. Day one of our first patient: day one of learning how to take apart a human.

III.

My neighbor is 87 years old, the age my anatomical donor was when he died. Sometimes I look at my neighbor and wonder what his body looks like on the inside, what's going wrong with it, and what he'll end up dying of. Sometimes I look at other people, or myself in the mirror, and wonder what our bodies look like on the inside, what's going wrong inside us, what we'll die of, and when. Sometimes I also look at people (strangers, mostly) and begin to take their bodies apart in my mind: wondering which of their body parts is malfunctioning, and why, like a guessing game of matching the stranger with the diagnosis. I don't mean patients who come to clinical settings, where it's then my job to try and figure out what's wrong. I mean people who haven't asked me anything, people who may have no bodily complaints at all, people I don't even know. That woman sitting next to me on the bus, or that man walking past the café. People going about their days, with the right to their privacy about their bodies. And yet, I can't help it. I analyze the way their fingers lie, the way their knees turn, the way their jaws move. I see these body parts in isolation, a hand here and a leg there, before even considering what these people are like as human beings. I fake-diagnose them by their body parts: the woman on the bus might have Marfan Syndrome; the man by the café may have Parkinson's. The thoughts come against my will. I diagnose diseases these strangers probably don't have and would likely want kept secret if they did. I'm not sure which is better: mentally giving a stranger a fake disease that she's lucky to not actually have or identifying her real disease without permission. Both make me cringe, and yet I transgress nonetheless.

In medical school, I am learning a sacred form of knowledge: the ability to read people's bodies to understand things about them that sometimes they do not yet know themselves. I wonder how I can train my mind to only do so when it's appropriate, to keep my knowledge sacred, and not to slip into the profane.

IV.

In the medical world, prenatal technology—such as ultrasound devices—by its nature means that we first visualize unborn humans as body parts. Last week, I saw a 22-week fetus inside the womb of a woman elated about her pregnancy. The physician moved the ultrasound device back and forth, and the mother stared in blissful wonder, part-by-part, watching her fetus come into view: here's a hand and a foot; here's a nose, an eye, a chin; here's a tibia, a fibula, a scapula, a spine. Meet your baby. (Or at least these parts will become your healthy baby. We hope.)

I have also been inside the room for an abortion, in which a physician similarly examined a fetus part-by-part, first by ultrasound and later by petri dish. Parts to be counted, to make sure nothing was left. I did not previously know that a fetus must be examined by parts to make sure it no longer exists. I support the mother's decision to end her pregnancy. I understand and welcome that the mother, not the fetus, is my patient. And yet, nonetheless, counting the body parts in the dish, assembling a would-be human that way, shook me. Those miniature hands, floating there in the dish—who knew they would look so perfect? How, and when, do parts of a human become a whole?

V.

It's March, which means we've been dissecting cadavers for eight months now, and I've been a medical student for the same amount of time. Hello again, "group 5-2" anatomy donor. In these past eight months, we've looked at your heart and your lungs, your viscera, and your vessels. Today we are looking at your brain. It's gray and grooved, about the weight and size of a large potato. It's smaller than it once was, likely from both the preservation methods and the Alzheimer's Disease that the paper taped to the wall says you died with. With your brain removed, the inside of your skull is shaped like a bowl, smooth but with canals where your brain and its vessels lay. Your skull shimmers with pale pinks and blues, iridescent like an abalone shell. Ethereal, beautiful colors I haven't seen anywhere else in your gray body, colors I didn't know could come from inside a human.

What surprised you, in your life? As a child, what gave you joy—was it flying your first kite, eating ice cream in the sun? What about as an adult—what was it that gave you so much joy you hurt with the realization that someday it must go away? What was it that crushed you with sadness, made you feel that you couldn't move, couldn't breathe? And how is it possible you're gone and yet also still here: how is it possible I'm standing in this stained lab coat holding your brain in the palm of my hand?

Donor, despite the bustle of the other anatomy students surrounding me, as I hold your brain in my hand, I feel alone in the universe. Learning to see people as bodies can feel so isolating—isolating from my former self, isolating from my friends and family, isolating from my spirituality. Yet the clock ticks, and I have clinic right after lab, which means there is no time for existential thoughts or emotions. It takes all my willpower to let those go, to focus instead on finishing the lab by investigating the parts of your body: locate your foramen magnum, identify your hypoglossal nerve.

Our lab instructor informs us that to make space on the table, we're permitted to remove your heart, lungs, and other organs (examined in previous dissections) and put them in your body bucket for cremation. We look down at the bucket, up at each other, and collectively decide we would prefer to keep your organs inside your body. But with your abdomen now gaping open, your organs partially spill out no matter how we position you. Rather than truly inside you, they're now on the edge between inside and outside, preserved in liminality. Where are the boundaries of your body?

I notice that the tag on your ear—the one stamped with your body number and "University of Michigan"—also says something else in the same small block letters: "Body, whole." Somehow it took me until today, when your body has become barely recognizable as a body, to see those words.

VI.

I deliberately start my days with lungs now, sitting on a cushion and focusing on my breath before making coffee or turning on my phone. Breathe through the whole lung space. Breathe in, breathe out. Observe thoughts and sensations. Label them, let them go. At a leadership training that came with free coffee cake, I made a commitment to doing this morning meditation for 49 days. And yet, it helps, taking these deep, purposeful breaths. It feels good to start the day this way. Maybe I don't mind seeing myself as a walking pair of lungs. Maybe that's all any of us are.

But I'm making an unfair claim: with healthy lungs, it's easy for me to label myself as a walking pair of lungs. It's easy for us to accept identity in the parts of us that are healthy.

Boundless Thanks to My Past Selves

Hadrian Kinnear

I was 10 years old and standing on the pitcher's mound on an early September day. I had butterflies in my stomach when my coach pulled me from first base to put me in as pitcher in the middle of a softball game. I'd been learning along with several others, but certainly did not feel ready. I prayed that I wouldn't hit the batter. Taking a deep breath, I reminded myself that thinking about it too much would probably make it more likely I would hurt someone. It was a learning process then, and I can't say that pitching ever became my strongest position. But for a shy kid who was suddenly the center of attention, working through those insecurities made other brave steps easier to take.

The year I turned 20, I set out alone to hike the Appalachian Trail from Maine to Georgia. For five months and ten days, I steadily back-packed 2,190 miles, carrying only the essentials on my back and wearing through several pairs of boots. Some in my community worried that the hike was simply too much to take on and did not understand why I felt called to embark on it. I vividly remember a late September evening spent on the trail in a Virginia hostel, sharing a communal meal with several other thru-hikers. After dinner, we sat around a cozy fire and tried to explain to some other guests at the hostel why we all felt compelled to put our lives on pause for months to hike.

I couldn't fully articulate my thoughts or feelings, but I felt grateful to be around other people who understood.

I came out as a transgender man at 25, early in my medical education. I knew then that living openly was risky, and I made a list of all of the things I was scared about losing: partner, family, school, community. Having not yet met any transgender physicians, I was particularly nervous about what this might mean for my career. One email to the entire medical school and many bureaucratic and emotional hurdles later, I made space for myself to exist authentically in all parts of my life.

Today, I climb onto my bike and feel the mid-morning sun of an unusually warm February on my back. As I pedal toward campus, my mind starts racing with thoughts about my clinical rotations, which will begin in a week. I'm about to start applying my insufficient knowledge to patients in the hospital, and I expect I will feel out of place most of the time. I'm not yet sure what this will look like for me, but I have heard that these upcoming rotations have a way of humbling everyone. I take several deep breaths, feel the wind rushing by me, and remind myself that I will be okay.

My 10-year-old self appears as I prepare to walk into the operating room in a week. I remind myself that thinking about all of the things I could do wrong might not be the most productive train of thought. I'm still shy. I still don't want to be the center of attention, and I'm not looking forward to getting yelled at if I'm in the way or if I bump into something important. The stakes are higher now than softball pitching, but the feeling is oddly similar—excitement about trying something new, mixed with the fear of letting people down and hurting someone.

As I try to explain my new schedule to my non-medical community (wake up at 4 a.m., bike to the hospital, hopefully be home before bedtime, get 24 hours "off" each week), I feel like my 20-year-old self explaining a thru-hike. Both the thru-hike and medical school are deeply solo journeys in the context of a community. In both settings, I often learn and draw strength from those around me, but ultimately, my progress remains my responsibility. During medical school, I have gathered around bonfires with friends and classmates to reflect on our experiences. Much like when I shared stories around the fire at the hostel in Virginia, I have had a similar feeling of not quite being able to explain why I feel called to this career but blessed to be around other people who understand.

As I prepare to be a trans medical student in a clinical setting, I feel more grounded and ready to be present with my patients and colleagues as a fully integrated person. My work and leadership are easier, and my community has offered love and support in response to my vulnerability. I hope my time in medical school and doing research will allow me to pay it forward and enrich the lives of others coming after me.

For me, each time I had to take a leap of faith, I have tried to listen to the part of me that had some inkling of the direction that my future self might appreciate. Each decision and moment of growth has had its insecurities and risks, and I have tried to persist in spite of the butterflies in my stomach. Looking back today, as I prepare to start my clinical rotations, I want to give boundless thanks to my past selves for their courage. They've set me up well, and I fully expect to draw strength from these memories in the coming weeks in clinic.

Consumed

Anonymous

JD is a 52-year-old woman with a history of diabetes and depression presenting with right upper quadrant pain.

Despite my progress, the word "depression" is all it takes, and any learning I was supposed to glean from this case discussion abruptly grinds to a halt. My first two years of medical school have helped me to intellectualize the effect of trauma on the brain, sure, to picture my hypertrophied amygdala and imagine the powerful neuronal pathways reinforced daily. But this does little to bring me comfort. Listening to so many case presentations during medical school has made it difficult not to imagine myself as the patient, and my mind now wanders to creating my own History of Present Illness—a concise summary of a patient's presentation.

Patient is a 25-year-old woman with a history of sexual trauma and family history of depression presenting with intrusive thoughts and panic symptoms.

I notice my hands are shaking and place them beneath the table so my classmates don't notice. How can they understand that my mind, simultaneously my greatest asset and enemy, is not my own? That my body is not my own. That I am both a girl who is, and a girl who was? I am here in the classroom, but I am not: I am in a white room, on a white couch, while men wearing golden chains smile down at me. I am being carried through the hallways of an unknown apartment building. I am hiding in a dark, metal staircase until it is safe to run. I am alone, in my bedroom, as my friends slowly stop leaving food outside my door, then stop coming around altogether. It has been five years now since that warm Wednesday in July when I was raped during my college semester abroad, but it still lingers, still festers and smolders, right beneath the surface. That is something no one told me about sexual assault—you never really get over it, you just learn to live with it. As you begin to move through your regular life after being so callously used and violated, every interaction feels exhaustingly rehearsed, like the curtain has been pulled back on the whole performance as friends transform into spectators. Then that life no longer feels familiar, and you start from scratch.

Social history is notable for polysubstance abuse, high-risk sexual behaviors, and alcoholism, which she tells herself is under control. Patient also struggles with how to share this part of her identity with her peers because, while overwhelming to her, this disability is entirely hidden. Physical exam is notable for tachycardia, hypertension, tachypnea, a slight tremor, and mydriasis.

As my classmates and faculty continue to discuss JD's predicament, I feel as if the room is filling with water and I am running out of air. So, I deploy my one weapon to prevent a public breakdown: I turn the volume dial on the outside world all the way down, retreating into myself while keeping my face perfectly slack. The past still emerges—I hear their laughter, see their eyes, smell cologne—but I appear at least as engaged as my classmates in the unfolding case discussion. I stare blankly at the incompletely erased whiteboard wall in front of me, the smudged and distorted reminders of the past. Suddenly, I hear a voice in my direction. I abruptly return to reality, unaware of how much of my time has been hijacked, and see that everyone is looking at me expectantly.

"I'm sorry, can you repeat that?" I mutter.

"What tests would you order on this patient?"

Collecting myself, I suggest liver function tests, then paradoxically chuckle and shake my head. Although the battle has subsided for now, it will return. How peculiar it is to live the life of both provider and patient.

Her biggest concern today is how she can, in theory, draw from her experiences as a powerful source of empathy. But she wonders how she can hope to support vulnerable people for a living when the slightest mention of mental health or abuse still condemns her to self-destruction.

For a long time, getting through each day felt so intolerable that my future was painted by fear and uncertainty. Although I am now at one of the best medical schools in the country, surrounded with opportunity, I still cyclically return to these moments of dread, most often in response to stress. Moving to Michigan was supposed to be a fresh start, but I never imagined how triggering the process of medical school would be. It is agonizing and exhausting confronting your inner demons in an academic context, bridging the extraordinarily intimate with the cool, calm, and collected persona of a physician. What do you do when you see so much of yourself in your patients? I was beginning to think I was out of the woods, but the flashbacks have become more frequent of late, stemming from a mix of triggering politicians, arrested sunlight, a difficult break-up, and—perhaps most frustratingly—the pre-clinical psychiatry course.

I thought I'd love the specialty. After all, I know all too well the influence of mind over every aspect of the body and the profound importance of having someone truly listen to your story. But instead, as I studied the discipline, and as the DSM-V read less like a textbook and more like a diary, my days began to spiral more into darkness and memories as I struggled to keep things impersonal. Reflecting on this, it seems that my desire to utilize my past to help others like me stands in direct opposition to my sanity. This instability is what scares me most about my upcoming third year of medical school, the year of the infamous grueling clinical rotations. I wonder how I will survive my clerkships, especially the psychiatry clerkship, when there is so much more to confront with less time to feel.

My leading diagnosis for this patient is Post-Traumatic Stress Disorder, supported by her experience of frequent flashbacks, nightmares, hyper-arousal, and feelings of isolation. Contributing to her diagnosis is an obsession with pleasing others, a complete lack of self-control, and a stubbornly unrealistic expectation for perfection. I am conflicted in terms of my plan for this patient. She endorses previous failed attempts to suppress, ignore, or drown these thoughts, but reports a steady improvement in her self-worth and quality of life over time. Despite valid concern over potential relapses, she is cautiously optimistic she will find a niche that bridges her multiple selves, enabling her to uniquely support others through life's inevitable obstacles.

I try my very best to not make my past into an excuse, to not let this define who I am. I am so many things: a survivor, yes, but also a daughter, sister, friend, artist, student, vivacious spirit, and healer. And yet, despite all of my development, all my strength, I frequently struggle with the influence and tenacity of that July Wednesday all those years ago. My future, my career, my relationship with my own mind, is uncertain: is it better for me to pursue a specialty that will offer distance and safety from it? Or, if I end up deciding to be a psy-chiatrist—if I vanquish the demons, debride the remaining disquiet, and find meaning in supporting victims of trauma and abuse—am I capitulating to my suffering? Am I allowing the events of a couple of hours too much influence over the arc of my life? Or, am I entering into a profession I am uniquely and intimately prepared to thrive in? I don't know.

But I do know that I have an extraordinary capacity to love, to live, and to learn, and that I cannot, will not, be again consumed.

All the Ward's a Stage

Hannah Cheriyan

There is something so comforting to me about a stage. Being given a role with defined parameters and knowing any mistakes I make won't affect the "real world" feels like a welcome release from the consequences of everyday life. Each year, our medical students write, perform, and direct an extravagant faculty roast in the form of a musical, dubbed "The Smoker." For the past two years, I have jumped enthusiastically into Smoker season. It's a cathartic process—not only a break from my textbooks, but a way to humorously acknowledge that there's more to medicine than memorizing medications. With a little song and dance, we can pose questions to the audience: "How do we get physicians to be more empathetic?"; "What's the best way to get doctors from different specialties to work together?"; and "Why are technology updates so difficult?" The magic, for me, is that we don't have to definitively answer these questions. We just explore them, offering a space to present ridiculous solutions and concerns that are just a little too valid for comfort.

Somehow, everything seems so much simpler when I'm on stage, looking out at the audience instead of sitting among them. Away from the stage, the choices I make matter in a more tangible fashion. As a pre-clinical student, my choices primarily affect me. A bad decision can be painful, but it's nothing in comparison to the sense of existential dread that comes with realizing soon my decisions will affect my patients. In the real world, we're dogged by Damocles' sword of choices: we can't afford to be wrong.

As nerve-racking as the world outside the theater can be, there isn't a complete separation between school and stage. Our class was the first in our school to take the new Doctoring course, where we met weekly with a small group of peers and two faculty mentors, learning the ins and outs of patient care. Going from our typical schedule of dry physiology lectures to brief but intense sessions rife with emotion—how to recognize child abuse, how to break the news that a patient has died—sometimes felt as if we were stepping into a whole different world. Our faculty mentors understood this and told us, "Treat this as a role, as a part you have to play. We'll practice until you know it well enough that it becomes instinctual."

For every part, there is a script to learn.

"What brings you in today?"

"Show me where the pain is."

"I understand why you're worried."

"We're going to do our best to get to the bottom of this."

For every part, there are stage directions.

Place your stethoscope at the left sternal border.

Extend the right leg until it is parallel to the ground.

Position the ophthalmoscope to visualize the retina.

When I started practicing patient interviews and physical exams, I felt flung into an overwhelming mass of clinical standards I didn't yet fully understand, so I clung tightly to my "scripts." Those "scripts" were both comforting and troubling. How could I be a real doctor if I was just mimicking my faculty mentors and rattling off checklists of symptoms? But as I became more comfortable with the words, I started to more fully understand why we used them and how to change my dialogue to make sure my audience—our standard-ized patients—understood the information I was trying to convey.

I learned to listen to cues from my patients to identify their fears and to extemporize descriptions of disease processes in layman's terms.

As with any rehearsal process, not everything went as planned in these practice patient scenarios. Sometimes I forgot entire sections of the physical exam or didn't ask the right questions and so completely missed the diagnosis. My classmates and I were especially error-prone when we practiced breaking bad news, too taken aback by the emotional outbursts of the actors playing our patients to respond as thoughtfully as we should have. But at each mistake, our faculty mentors would gently talk us through what went wrong and how we could improve. They revealed errors they had made during their own careers as physicians, and they emphasized the importance of owning your mistakes and telling the patient, "I'm sorry." In a safe space where both our peers and our mentors could share their vulnerabilities, clinical responsibilities seemed more manageable. True, the Doctoring course was just rehearsal for the "opening night" of our upcoming years as clinical students, but it helped to know that our eventual performances wouldn't always have to be perfect.

Soon, our class will be entering the wards. In a few days, I will test how well I can identify with my patients and how well I can communicate in a language they understand. I know I will probably feel out of place and unsure of my "role" as my rotations begin. But I also know, in times like this, I can turn to the nurturing of the theater and the lessons our faculty mentors taught us.

I am ready for the curtain to rise.

Clinical Essays

Heartbreak

Hsin (Cindy) Lee

From heart to hand to head and back to heart. Heartbroken in agony, with a pull of a trigger, his brain was lost—broken like his heart, but irreparably so. Less than 48 hours prior, he had ended his life, and I was there to witness as this meant giving life for someone else.

I had the opportunity to be on the Transplant service during my surgery rotation as a third-year medical student. I had heard joining for an organ procurement is the pinnacle of the transplant experience. It was the last night of my time on service, and I hadn't participated in a procurement yet. I wasn't officially on the schedule to be on call, but as I packed up my stuff for the afternoon, my senior resident asked, "If we get a procurement tonight, do you want me to let you know?"

I answered, "Absolutely."

At 9 p.m., my pager went off: "Procurement tonight. Scheduled for 12 a.m. You in?" I put my scrubs back on and headed back to the hospital. I got to the team room in University Hospital to start reading about the donor. The organ donor was Sam, a young man who had taken his own life through a self-inflicted gunshot wound to the head.

I felt a lump in my throat as my breath caught. I had to take a deliberate, deep breath as I continued to read through the Emergency Room note from the attending physician, then from the social worker, then the clergy. They had each added details as to what had led Sam from being a healthy, seemingly happy young man to someone acutely suffering from self-disappointment and heartbreak, to an organ donor pronounced brain dead a few hours ago.

I had been so focused on the excitement of getting to join for a procurement, thinking, "Wow, am I lucky! This is my last night on service!" I hadn't paused to think at all about the meaning of this yet. I still, undeniably, felt eager in the sense that I was curious to learn, but my feelings were no longer one-dimensional. I felt my enthusiasm begin to intermix with feelings I couldn't really name yet as I started to realize the depth of meaning for the lives involved in this case. But I quickly put those feelings away, gathered my belongings from the team room, and walked over to meet up with my senior resident before the start of the case.

The Operating Room (OR) was ready. We waited in the hallway for Sam to arrive. He arrived covered in a colorful, fleece tie-blanket, clearly from home. I was surprised for a few seconds to not see him arrive in off-white, industrial-appearing blankets like all the other patients I had seen en route from pre-op to the OR. Then I realized that, unlike every other patient I saw on surgery, Sam didn't arrive alive. What else would be more important than making sure he remained surrounded by a representation of love and comfort for as long as possible?

It was becoming more difficult to keep my feelings at bay.

Following the team's confirmation of the patient's identity and plan for operation, we all took a moment of silence. Then the surgery began. Sam would be donating his kidneys, liver, and pancreas. The first two hours went by quickly and calmly as the senior resident and fellow carefully dissected out and identified the relevant anatomy. It was a rare and valuable teaching opportunity in anatomy as the fellow asked me to name the parts they diligently isolated, especially because (excepting the fact that he was brain dead) Sam was entirely healthy. His organs were un-diseased—beautiful almost—the closest to Netter's[1] I think could reasonably be expected. We carried on, naming vessels and landmarks, until it was time to turn our attention to the heart.

Sam had gone into cardiac arrest before being declared brain dead, making his heart ineligible for donation. The plan was to vent the right atrium and flush the heart.

The fellow asked me, "Ready?"

A suction in each hand, I nodded my head. "Ready."

The fellow punctured the right atrium, and I suctioned away the blood as it rushed out of the wound. For the next 30 minutes, I stood amazed, mesmerized, shocked, disturbed by the struggle. I was awed by the Heart's stubbornness to just keep trying to do its job despite the fact that it was dying. The fellow told me to look up at the EKG. The anesthesiologist turned the screen toward me.

"A. fib," he said. I quickly looked up.

"Ah, I see." Then my eyes flew back to the Heart.

It was beating even harder, as if it could get a head start and outrun the life-ending injury it had just sustained. Its ventricles flexed to compensate for its wound like a man with his pectoral muscles puffed out to compensate for his insecurities. But the Heart's insecurity could not be hidden. The blood continued to pour out, and despite its attempt to puff out its chest, it was shrinking as the volume carrying life flooded out. And I stood there, sucking it all away with two white plastic suctions.

"V. tach."

"Right."

Eyes back to the Heart, the struggling Heart.

As his Heart became rapidly lighter, mine rapidly became heavier. All the feelings I had been deliberately putting away came down on me hard as I felt the weight of what I was witnessing as well as the

---

1   Referring to the *Atlas of Human Anatomy* by Frank H. Netter, MD

hot, salty tears flowing down my face. I didn't even know what I was feeling yet. I just knew I was terribly sad.

The Heart's stubbornness afforded me the time to get over the shock, and my mind went back to Sam. Did he struggle before his death the same way his heart struggled before its death? Before he pulled the trigger that ended his life, was his heart racing to make up for the lost beats it would never have?

My thoughts turned to Sam's family. I was standing here next to him. Where were they? "Devastated" seems like a sorry understatement for what his mom must have been feeling over the past 48 hours. I remembered the chart note I read back in the team room: "When this volunteer visited patient's room, patient's little brother lying in bed next to patient." The tears seemed to be pouring out now. It was getting difficult to keep my breaths regular, as I was trying not to be noticed.

"V. fib," the fellow said, bringing my thoughts away from Sam and back to the Heart. I didn't look up at the EKG for that one. I couldn't take my eyes away from the Heart. I could see through my annoyingly pervasive tears that the muscles in the atria were no longer synced up with the ventricles. What if my stream of tears broke sterility? Was I going to contaminate the surgical field with my uncontrollable emotion? Why couldn't I stop crying?

There was something about watching the Heart that made the fact that a life had ended undeniably real, and it forced upon me a raw appreciation for the gravity of the life and death of transplantation. Seeing the Heart pump strongly, then slowly progress to pumping even harder, then asynchronously, then finally lose its endurance and decline until its remaining movements were a random quiver here and there in the right atrium was intensely emotional. Even before my mind consciously started mourning for Sam's life, his family's pain, and the miraculous and strange fact that I was watching and participating as the blood drained away from his organs in death,

I knew they would soon refill with someone else's to bring a new chance at life. Yet, before these thoughts could come together, there was something visceral, something inherently and profoundly sad about watching the Heart break.

I had so many emotions, many of which I still don't really know what to call, but two of which were humility and gratitude. As my thoughts and emotions raced between the Heart, Sam, the family, the surgeons, the EKG, the recipient, and at some point, myself, I vividly wondered: who am I to be the one standing here, watching something so personal and meaningful? I felt an odd mixture of appreciation and self-consciousness, realizing this was not something many people would experience, yet here I was. Should I have been there in this remarkably private and deeply significant moment for Sam and his family? I silently hoped my tears and emotions were some sort of homage to Sam and his family, and though tiny and unknown to them, these would make it okay that I was present in this most intimate and final moment.

Unbolting the Gate of Locked-In Syndrome

Gabrielle Shaughness

Obtaining a broad, general exposure to the various medical special-ties is the objective of the third year of medical school. As we rotate through the various fields, some disciplines may be more interesting than others. It can require mindfulness to regard each day—even the days when one is rotating through a field one has no intention of pursuing—as gifts. Every morning, as I ride my bicycle to the hospi-tal, knowing that God does not waste a single day of a person's life, I pray that God will enable me to do His work through the people and situations the day brings. Mr. B. is one of these people.

On the first day of my Neurology rotation, I followed the residents as we made our morning rounds to visit patients on the stroke unit. The residents asked the students to each choose a few patients we found interesting to follow for the duration of our rotation. When we came to Mr. B.'s room, he was lying in bed, unresponsive, a trache-ostomy tube in his neck. Mr. B. had suffered a brainstem stroke. He had been unresponsive for the past few days and was now showing possible signs of pneumonia. This combination of medical problems intimidated me as a student. Mr. B.'s case would be far over my head, I thought, and I crossed him off my list of potential patients to follow.

Every morning, the resident caring for Mr. B. updated the team about his condition in a tone increasingly stale and hopeless: Mr. B.

was "still unresponsive, no change." The resident would attempt a brief neurologic exam, but as Mr. B. could neither move nor speak, I started to sense the resident was merely performing the exam as a required exercise, without much hope that his findings would change.

Later that week, the resident notified us we would need to choose one patient for a teaching rounds demonstration with a neuro-ophthalmologic specialist. We didn't have any patients who had any eye symptoms in particular so the resident resigned, "I guess you can use Mr. B., but he is not very interesting because he can't do anything."

Underwhelmed with our not-very-interesting patient, we presented Mr. B.'s history. The attending physician then began his physical exam, proceeding slowly and deliberately to teach us a thorough neurological assessment. His level of attention and care stood in stark contrast to the rushed exam I had observed on rounds every morning. When asked to squeeze the attending's hand, Mr. B. showed no reaction, as usual.

"Can you raise your eyebrows?" the attending continued. "No? How about, can you wiggle your toes? As hard as you can, come on, give us a good effort." With one command after the next, he was unable to demonstrate any movement or awareness.

Finally, the attending asked, "Mr. B., close your eyes. Good. Now, if you can understand me, open your eyes." Mr. B. opened his eyes wide. But perhaps this was just coincidence, as people in a vegetative state can demonstrate spontaneous eye movements. To verify, the attending spent the next five minutes probing with concrete "yes" or "no" questions to which he asked Mr. B. to blink his eyes accordingly.

It suddenly became clear to all of us that this response was no coincidence.

I had to fight back tears when the attending asked in conclusion, "Mr. B., do you consider yourself to be paralyzed?"

Two blinks—"yes"—confirmed our growing suspicion that, although he was unable to move any part of his body except his eyelids, he was cognitively completely intact, his mind held prisoner in a body that could not respond.

"This is a very rare condition," the attending explained to his audience of residents and students, "one that you will never forget because it is devastating—'locked-in syndrome.'"

Later that afternoon, I returned to Mr. B.'s room on my own. The gravity of the situation had started to hit me as I felt overwhelmed with guilt that we had all written Mr. B. off as a "vegetable." How scared and frustrated he must have been all this time to not be able to speak or move, unable to tell us, "I am here! I am trapped in my own body. Please do not abandon me!"

I took Mr. B.'s hand in my own and, being sure we were alone, I apologized to him as I fought back my tears.

"I didn't know you were there," I cried, "I'm so, so sorry this happened to you."

Then, with great hesitation because I was nervous about overstepping boundaries as a member of the medical team, I ventured, "Mr. B., I am going to ask you a personal question. If it offends you or you do not want me to discuss it further, then just close your eyes— 'no'—and I will immediately drop it. Mr. B., is faith an important part of your life?"

He opened his eyes wide—"Yes."

Given my fear of agitating him, his positive response was a relief. To be certain I was not misinterpreting his eye blinks, I verified with a few more questions. Once assured that God was important to him, I squeezed his hand again in mine and whispered, "I am going to pray for you. And I want you to remember, even if none of the rest of us can hear you because you are trapped in there, you can pray to God, because He can hear you."

Tears started rolling down Mr. B.'s face. I quickly became nervous that I was upsetting Mr. B. so I again asked him to respond with eye blinks if he wanted me to be quiet and leave. But he blinked for me to stay and keep talking.

I spent the rest of the afternoon and that week talking to Mr. B. Using just "yes" or "no" eye movements, I found out which musicians he enjoyed. Our occupational therapist was able to get an iPad for him, onto which we downloaded these favorite musicians and set a timer to automatically shut off after an hour. "Do you want to listen to music today? Blink 'Yes,' if so."

One afternoon, as I was leaving, I saw someone with a strong resemblance to Mr. B. standing outside his room. I introduced myself and excitedly started explaining the eye-blinking method of communication we had devised as well as some of the preferences Mr. B. had "told" me.

"He likes the same music as I do, even the gospel group 'The Blind Boys of Alabama.'"

"Well, that's because he is a pastor," Mr. B's brother replied.

Stunned, I stuttered, "So all this time I was nervous to pray aloud because I didn't want to get in trouble if anyone overheard me, and you're telling me I was praying with a pastor?"

As medical professionals, we refrain from sharing details of our personal lives as we strive to focus completely on the lives of our patients. We learn to filter our own emotions to remain neutral; perhaps our personal opinions may offend the patient before us. Thus, we sterilize not only our tools but our demeanor as well. This bleaching of our personal passions, particularly with regards to faith, has troubled me. God is so central to my purpose in my work that I want to celebrate Him, discuss Him, and share Him with all those I meet. My career means little to me if it is not used to glorify God by being a tool of His grace and mercy in caring for people.

Unsolicited sharing of this passion, however, can greatly offend strangers in my care who do not share the same faith. Given that the priority is on the patient's needs and not my own, I find myself treading cautiously in a professional setting as I struggle with the repressed yearning to share and encourage others in Christ. I also wonder whether withholding inquiry into another's soul sometimes deprives our patient of a type of healing that, at times, may be the only treatment left when our scalpels and drugs can do no more. We are trained not to fear cutting a person's chest open, yet we often avoid unpacking the role faith plays in our patient's life. I have not yet reconciled the tension I feel in balancing professional versus personal priorities in my patient interactions, but I've been trying to gauge when I might be able to step a bit closer to the personal side, as I did with Mr. B.

The friendship between me and Mr. B. was unexpected—he an elderly man and I a young woman, communicating with each other using only the blink of his eyes, connected through our mutual love for Christ. We cried together that first afternoon when I realized he was cognitively intact as he lay motionless in his bed, his tears his only method of responding as we prayed. We rejoiced together in good ol' Southern gospel music. He will never be able to speak a word to me, but with his eyes alone, we have had conversations that have brought us into fellowship as children of God.

As I shared his story with friends and loved ones, I saw tears of joy on their faces or heard sighs of awe over the telephone. Some even told me they had gone on to retell his story to their own family and, in doing so, Mr. B. had brought encouragement to people he would never meet. Taking these responses back to Mr. B., I held his hand as I looked in those thoughtful, wise eyes of his and said, "It may not have occurred to you, paralyzed as you are in this hospital bed, but I want you to know you continue to minister to people you don't even know clear across the country. I know you wish you could still preach on Sunday and speak aloud of God's love, but even from the silence of this bed, know that people are hearing of how God has been working in this room, showing His grace and comfort through the inspiration you have brought me. Even though you may not be able to speak, people are hearing your story. You are still preaching, Mr. B., still preaching."

The Gallbladder Isn't Green

Daniel Nelson

I chose surgery as the first clerkship of my clinical years very deliberately. I was almost certain I didn't want to pursue it as a career, and
I figured I had little to lose by getting it out of the way quickly.
It meant I would experience at the outset what my peers regarded as
the most time-intensive rotation, thus making the hectic demands of
the remainder of the year somewhat tamer in comparison. I admit
I entered the rotation biased and a bit wary about how the surgeons
would treat us as students, my mind filled with the stereotypes of
tyrants with scalpels. And I will also admit, in nearly every case,
I was proven wrong by dedicated surgeons who were invested in my
learning. This extended from early-career faculty members to the
most powerful figures in the department. It was, in my observation,
almost uniform for the surgeons to treat us well.

Almost. During my first time in the operating room—the hallowed
OR—I was with a surgeon performing a rather extensive operation.
I knew the physician I would be working with had academic interests
similar to mine, so I figured the two of us would have a connection
beyond our arbitrary pairing. He was the surgeon I was least nervous
to be with in the OR. Why was I so interested in who was operating?
Medical education is defined by its traditions, with the practice of
"pimping" central among them. The pimper—the questioner, and in
my case, the surgeon I operated with—asks questions in something
resembling the Socratic method, though with the additional objective

of subjugating the person being pimped. Pimp questions are almost always asked of someone of lesser academic rank. Friendly attending physicians ask questions that are either easy or good-natured enough to defuse this hierarchical tension; this technique makes pimping a genuinely helpful educational tool. However, less kindly educators can be ruthless.

I was advised by fellow students and the residents on our team that, for every surgery, I needed to prepare in advance by reading up on the operation, the underlying disease, and the patient's medical history. Despite this guidance, I could hardly guess what I might be asked. And beyond trying to answer pimp questions correctly, I wanted to be engaged in the operation, asking well-informed questions of my own to demonstrate my deep reading and interest. (The unengaged student appears more vulnerable to the predatory pimper.)

The night before the surgery I read as much as I could to prepare. I read about the outcomes of the surgery, including surgery-related mortality rates, post-surgery prognosis, typical complications, and recovery time. I read about the diagnosis and natural history of the patient's underlying condition. I read about my patient's initial presentation and her medical comorbidities. I looked up the relevant body structures and the steps of the operation, manipulating in my mind the images I saw on the pages of my anatomy text until my eyelids sagged.

I entered the OR with trepidation, even knowing I was well-prepared. But not long into the operation, I was lost. The anatomy of the abdomen looked entirely different from how it did in Netter's Anatomy and different from the cadavers I'd dissected during my anatomy courses. Occasionally, I recognized something and could reorient myself, though I would, in short order, become confused again. I was treading anatomical water, but I tried asking a question or two to show the surgeon I was engaged and, clearly, not lost. During one of my subsequent moments of disorientation, I noticed the surgeon was removing a white, glossy structure from near the liver. I remembered a part of the procedure involved cutting down one of the liver's attachments to the body wall, so I wondered if that was the structure I saw. I felt this was a good time for a question:

"What is that structure you are removing?" I asked, hoping—though with some confidence—that I was on the right track.

The surgeon stopped, looked up at me, and said, "The gallbladder." He continued, tersely, "You know, if you really want to learn, you need to make sure you read about the operation we are performing in advance. Otherwise you are just wasting your time in here. You can't expect to come in unprepared and get anything out of it."

The schoolchild's hand of my intellect had been slapped. I wished I wasn't there—grateful for the refuge of a surgical mask. I *had* read about the operation and had done so fairly vigorously, so I thought. But I had never seen a gallbladder *in vivo*; every anatomy book I had read colored it an earthy green, which correlated well with the specimens of the gallbladder from my dissection labs. The bile it concentrates apparently stains its walls—but only after death. The thin, cream-colored structure I saw him working with was not at all familiar. A bit ashamed, I told myself I should have known what it was and moved on.

After that, I prepared even more fiercely in advance of working with him, certain I could demonstrate my talent. Despite my efforts, even the best questions I posed to him yielded short, one-word responses. When he asked me questions, I carefully replied, certain there would be a reprisal of our first time in the OR together. Instead, my answers were met with silence. On one occasion, tired of not knowing whether my answers were right or wrong, I asked if I had been correct—a reasonable request, since, after all, medical school is for learning.

His response? "No."

I still don't know where that structure gets its blood supply. I hated feeling so ashamed.

Tragically, this surgeon was once a new clinical student like me, trembling behind his own surgical mask. Yet he produced the sort of environment he had dreaded. Every physician has endured volleys of pimp questions during their training, though the usefulness of the practice when applied in the style of this surgeon is questionable. Better put, the *educational* usefulness of pimping like this is questionable. Sure, it has had plenty of use as a tool for generations of physicians to inculcate an apparently proper fear of student for teacher. But despite their historical predominance, this breed of physician is becoming rarer. I have met a handful or two of kind, talented educators for every person like my first surgeon-teacher on the faculty, and I expect the balance will continue to tip this way. Medical education is likely to grow friendlier and, I think, more effective, however gradually it changes. In the meantime, medical students should remember to endure the barbs of these physician-teachers with the knowledge that we all have taken them—and of course, remember that the gallbladder isn't *actually* green.

The Line

Meredith Hickson

I walk to morning rounds under the covered walkways that con-
nect the hospital's freestanding wards. I feel the daily rhythm of this
place hum to life as I pass the meadow where patients' family members spent the night and are now folding their mats and blankets.
They light charcoal braziers to boil tea and flour for porridge. They
haul water from the public tap to wash their loved ones' bed linens.
The public hospital provides no meals, no bedding, and no nursing care beyond what is necessary to change bandages and adminis-
ter medications. What the hospital has, it provides for free: a thinly
stocked pharmacy; a few aging lab machines; and a small staff of
dedicated, resourceful general practitioners, nurses, and midwives.
What it lacks—an obstetrician and pediatrician, x-ray and ultrasound
machines, a ventilator, and many essential medicines—is often the
cause of death for the impoverished patients who cannot afford a
better-equipped, private hospital.

I reach the children's ward just as rounds start. The intern and
chief nurse begin with a young woman seated on one of the beds
packed end-to-end into the narrow room. She is holding an infant
who is smaller than he should be. The skin of his face and chest,
exposed between the layers of blanket, is loose and pewter-gray. The
whites of his eyes are yellow. His mouth hangs open, and he gags
repeatedly. His mother brought him here because he has been vomiting incessantly for the past week, unable to breastfeed. On exam, his

mouth is coated with a thick, green thrush that travels past his tongue, down the back of his throat.

The chief nurse quickly diagnoses pyloric stenosis, a narrowing of the stomach that causes excessive vomiting in newborns. The intern—a sharp, compassionate woman whom I deeply respect—cautiously agrees. They make a plan to rehydrate the baby while they wait for laboratory results to come back. The intern scribbles in the composition book that serves as the boy's medical record and calls for a nursing student to insert an IV. The intern and the chief nurse start moving toward the next bed. I am slow to follow. There is a long list of possible diagnoses for a jaundiced, vomiting infant. The tests we've ordered will help pare it down, but I think we should test for something that neither the nurse nor the intern mentioned.

My role on the ward is poorly defined. I am a research fellow at the study center on the hospital grounds. The hospital superintendent placed no limits on my involvement in care. But an American physician collaborating on the same research study that brought me here told other American students and residents that, for reasons both ethical and legal, they were not permitted to express clinical opinions, make clinical suggestions, or interview patients. I quickly came to understand the purpose of these restrictions. The intern does not yet have a license to practice, and rounds are rarely attended by a senior physician. I am often asked directly by staff or patients to intervene in care because they believe a foreigner in a white coat can provide free care, or different care, or better care, than the hospital's own care team. If I suggest something inappropriately invasive, it might well be ordered anyway. If I involve myself, I risk dangerously exceeding the limits of my clinical knowledge.

So I have stuck to asking questions. I am here to learn, and the general practitioner who visits the ward once a week enjoys teaching. He is an excellent clinician, and I've seen him diagnose even rare, complex conditions on physical exam and experience alone. (These diagnoses are confirmed later at private hospitals with better labo-ratories.) Drug stock-outs, equipment failures, and the absence of a surgeon with pediatric training often prevent the staff from providing the necessary care, but, before today, I have never witnessed anything I suspected to be an error.

The staff are usually quick to consider HIV when a child who appears chronically ill arrives on the ward. I have seen the general practitioner order HIV testing for children in better shape than the boy we just examined. I don't know why the chief nurse and the intern chose not to.

I want to take the intern out of earshot to ask, but I hesitate. Conflicting ideas about what I have ethical license to do here, and the utter lack of supervision, hold me back. As I stand over her son, the mother begins to look concerned. Screening for HIV here starts with the mother. If she is positive, the child is tested. She told us there are other children at home. If this boy is positive, one or more of her other children might be as well, so I conclude HIV is worth at least asking about. I take the intern aside. I try to make it sound like academic curiosity and not a recommendation. I can tell that omit-ting the HIV serology was not intentional. She tells the chief nurse that we should order the test. He is her senior here, and running the ward is his responsibility.

The chief nurse, confident in his diagnosis of pyloric stenosis, does not see the necessity. He impatiently reminds the intern that we test women for HIV in pregnancy. To make his point, he loudly asks the boy's mother about the results of her prenatal test. Immediately, all other conversations in the room slow and then stop. Every adult pres-ent turns to face the mother and hear her reply. "Negative," she tells him almost inaudibly, her head down. The intern and I exchange a concerned look; anyone would lie when asked like this. Persistent, harsh stigma about HIV is a reality here, especially for women. The baby's mother knows this, even if the chief nurse does not.

The intern shifts her eyes from me to the chief nurse and back to me, anxiously. The chief nurse has seniority, and he is a man—a recipe for misery in any hospital hierarchy. The intern will not argue with him, and she will not order the test unless he agrees with her plan. However, this same chief nurse is quick to defer decisions to me, though I have so far declined to make any. Like the intern, I am younger and a woman, but I am also a foreigner with a stethoscope. If I second the intern's assessment, the boy will get tested.

A cool damp starts collecting on my palms and between my shoulders. This is why other students were warned not to get involved. Having a student's opinion and presenting a recommendation with the authority of a licensed physician are two very different things. Suddenly, I am standing on the line between studying medicine and practicing it, and I do not have permission to cross. Three long, rigorous years of acculturation to the world of medicine pin my tongue to the floor of my mouth; unsupervised students do not order tests. It doesn't matter that this is just a vial of blood. There is no fully trained doctor present to make the call, and it would be unethical to give myself that authority.

The boy's mother tries to breastfeed him. He cries weakly and gags. Physicians are trained to ask themselves a basic question when they see a new patient for the first time: is this person's condition likely to deteriorate further, or is it stable? In hospital-speak: sick or not sick? The answer depends largely on the intuition of experience. The more time I spend on the wards, the more comfortable I feel picking out the patients who need immediate attention. This baby's body is limp and hot. The skin between the open bones of his skull is so sunken with dehydration that I can see its depth before I feel it. His chest rises and falls rapidly, and his rib cage and belly suck in when he draws air; he is struggling to breathe. Sick, very sick.

It will be days before the general practitioner reviews the boy's case. The hospital's few physicians are responsible for hundreds of patients, spread out across many buildings. I have followed the care of children who died before a doctor could even examine them. Without an intensive care unit, we can do very little for an acutely ill child beyond providing IV fluids, and the staff can't refer him to a bigger hospital without a physician's assessment. Another lesson has been hammered home repeatedly: when you're stuck, start by looking for something you can treat. If the baby tests positive for HIV, at least the intern can start anti-retroviral drugs immediately and give antibiotics to treat and prevent opportunistic infections. It may not be enough, but it's far from nothing.

I remind myself, I shouldn't act like the doctor I'm not yet. Medicine is grounded in limits that protect patients and maintain confidence in physicians. But medicine is also about the patient in front of you, I tell myself, and I am not convinced that my staying on this side of the line is in his best interest.

"It couldn't hurt to re-check the prenatal clinic's results," I say. The chief nurse quickly agrees.

I walk home from the hospital along a red-dirt road that runs parallel to the paved one through town. I prefer the relative quiet of this route to the hectic evening traffic on the main road where motor-cycles loaded with three passengers (or two passengers and a goat… or one passenger and a massive, wobbly sack of charcoal…) swerve between cars and stray cattle. Brightly decorated public buses and trucks address the mayhem with dark humor—like "Don't Facebook, Face God"—stenciled on their bumpers.

In contrast, the dirt road passes through an area that indicates what life is like out of town. Corn and millet stalks grow thick on either side of the path and in dense rows between buildings, obscur-ing the mud-and-sheet-metal homes. Goats graze in culverts. Someone has planted sweet potatoes on a skinny strip of earth between a cement wall and the road. The economization of space here is desperate. These little urban subsistence farms aren't connected to the town water system or the grid. The baby in the children's ward and his mother are from a village that looks a lot like this but is even farther from town.

I think about how, no matter what the test results show, my involvement in that family's care may bring significant, unintended consequences for them. In a community as small as this one, the chances of gossip about the HIV conversation on the ward finding its way back to the mother's village are significant. By triggering a public discussion about her status, I might have caused her to be thrown out of her in-laws' home or fired from her job. Sometimes families disappear from the ward at night, overwhelmed by the impossible cost of care. I worry that this mother, overwhelmed by exposure, could also disappear.

Foreign healthcare providers have historically come with good intentions but assumed little or no liability for unintended consequences in places like this. I worked in a different country before medical school, and there I witnessed a particularly excessive example of such impunity. An American medical mission team arrived with the stated goals of training local doctors and providing much-needed care. In the course of their mission, however, they elected to forego informed consent and harmed or disabled multiple patients. On the day they left, they were thanked with gifts and a luncheon at the hospital's expense. Foreign researchers and clinicians who bring expertise, grant money, or equipment to a hospital in dire need, or who come from a country that aids the national healthcare system, may not face the same consequences they would at home, or the same consequences as the local staff, for failing to provide safe care.

A lack of accountability increases the inherent power differential between patients and physicians. Patient poverty further weights these relationships in favor of physicians. The disparity between this boy's family and me, a White woman, is widened by the history of colonialism here. Mothers on the ward tell their children I will eat them if they don't sit still for needle pricks. It's intended as a joke, for the adults at least, but it shows the long memory of foreign rule and the persistent association of Whiteness with violent authority.

Some have noted that academic global health resembles a second "scramble for Africa," with powerful, foreign universities carving out niches to extract data and provide learning opportunities for their own students. Few things sound more colonial than a White student getting away with something in a Black country that wouldn't fly at home. Except, perhaps, a student failing to prevent the death of a child because she has been trained to see his body and his country as a classroom in which her only obligation is to her own education.

That night, the intern texts me: "mom positive so we tested baby, also positive. both started on arvs."

Her message brings a flood of relief. If HIV does, in fact, explain all of the baby's symptoms, we may save his life, and we will certainly be able to help his mother. After initial counseling, community health workers will follow up with the family to ensure they receive their medications. I hope the medical benefits of testing will outweigh the social consequences. On medication, the boy has a long life expectancy. He'll be healthy enough to attend school in a few years. If, one day, he decides he wants to have a family, there are dating groups for positive singles and counseling for positive people who want to have children.

Then I remember his small, heaving chest and the nursing student frantically trying to insert an IV into his dry veins. The reality that he might be gone by the time we round tomorrow morning catches up to me.

At home, I never tried to protect myself from the possibility that a patient could die. I let myself invest. When we did lose a patient, I let myself feel the loss for as long as I needed. That felt like a healthy response, an emotionally honest response. I didn't realize until I got here how much the strength of my university teaching hospital shaped my behavior. We almost never lost a patient without a thorough fight. We had specialists to consult and an intensive care unit and experimental therapies to try. At the end, the family and the medical team knew everything possible had been done. Which meant that, while I often felt sad over the death of a patient, I almost never felt angry.

Here, anger feels like the emotionally honest response. I have followed the care of multiple children who died utterly irrational deaths—because there weren't enough staff, because we stocked out of antibiotics, because we ran out of blood to transfuse—deaths that make the real, statistical progress on childhood mortality in this country feel abstract. We can tell their parents we did everything we could, but we cannot tell them we did everything possible.

Anger, in the right dose, is motivating. In the wrong dose, it leads to ugly thoughts of futility. People who mentor students in settings like this are fond of saying that global health requires flexibility, patience, and creativity. No one has ever told me outright that it requires optimism. I guess that's assumed. Yet many people who spend long periods of time in places like the children's ward struggle with futility at some point. In my experience, not just optimism but *willful* optimism is necessary for students of global health. It checks futility; it balances anger. It helps me solve problems by reassuring me that there is, indeed, a solution. Idealism, an attitude that can result in rolling eyes back home, is also vital here. Optimism is the willingness to believe a way forward is possible. Idealism is a willingness to see the shape of the way. When it is my turn to be a mentor, I will encourage my students to cultivate both.

For the baby in the ward, I know that poverty and stigma still stand between him and his fifth birthday, but I choose to invest anyway. I choose to imagine the kind of childhood, the kind of adulthood, he could have. I choose to see that by protecting his mother's life, we have protected his. Global health is usually taught and discussed in terms of populations because the scope of both the challenges and the successes is so large. HIV is a prime example of both a massive challenge and an incredible success. Medicine, in any setting, is also about the patient in front of you. Zooming in from a population view to the view from the ground pushes me to reframe what works and what doesn't in terms of individual lives. Tomorrow, there will be new patients on the ward, and I will choose to see them not as case studies in HIV, malaria, or malnutrition, but as my patients.

It seems tempting now to shrug off how anxious I was about a simple blood test. I still don't feel comfortable, though, with my choice to steer care in a way in which students are not granted the ethical or legal authority to do back home. I remember the American surgeons I encountered during my last job in a hospital like this one. They ignored rules integral to the trust between patients and physicians because they knew they would not be held accountable. They serve as a warning to not only heed my uneasiness, but welcome it. I know now there will be other patients in the months ahead who force me to re-evaluate my role as a student. I don't know what I will do the next time I am faced with the line, but I hope it continues to force critical reflection and prompt self-restraint.

In a year, with scarcely more knowledge than I have right now, I will be a resident physician. Medical school trains us rigorously on how to make a plan, but responsibility for that plan is harder to teach. Training in environments like this hospital has been vital to learning what it means to be accountable for clinical decisions. Responsibility, as I interpret it now, cannot be a state of mind that switches on or off at the moment I am called upon to make a decision. Responsibility must be an active and ubiquitous awareness of the forces that shape who is invited to participate in deciding and the deep costs of the choice.

Recovery

Anitha Menon

She was dressed in black sweatpants and her red lacrosse t-shirt when she told us she wanted to die. I noticed scars under her sleeves. Our intake interview and initial interactions were uncomfortable. We listened with clinical distance when she mumbled the details of getting the knife she would use to kill herself. We listened when she told us she wouldn't make it to high school. We admitted Abby to the Child Psychiatry Unit for depression with suicidal ideation, plan, and intent. I'd seen her mother, dull from fatigue and worry, sitting in the waiting room earlier that morning. Her father was not there.

"He thinks I'm faking. Black people don't get depressed," she said, angry tears plastering her face.

It has been one week since she has been admitted, and he has not yet visited.

In the team room, the residents shake their heads at the father's behavior: *How could you treat your own daughter like that?* Objectively, it was appalling. What does it take for a parent to accept that their child has a mental illness? I nod passively, because I still don't know the answer to that question.

It took my own father 15 years just to acknowledge my anxiety. My father is a proud, stubborn, smart man who came to America by the grace of god and grit, with one pair of shoes, a young wife, and a baby daughter. No one in our Indian community had depression or anxiety (or rather, they did, but found it socially impolite to discuss).

To him, depression was the same as sadness, anxiety the same as worry. Both were rough patches you could lift yourself out of with enough determination. He dealt miserably with my anxiety. Or rather, he didn't deal with it at all, often stoking it with his own unchecked anger and impulsivity.

The first time I remember experiencing anxiety, I was 10 years old. I had a science competition project due the next morning and an oddly complicated idea: to build a musical instrument and play a piece on it. I had a) procrastinated greatly, beginning at 3 p.m. that afternoon, and b) gone horrifically overboard on my idea. I begged my dad to take me to Home Depot that night, as I dealt with the feelings associated with all the thoughts spinning around in my head: the shame of waiting so long to start a difficult project, the fear of the consequences, the shame again, the fear again. And, of course, there was the self-loathing, made no better by my dad's biting comments: *You need to grow up…you should have more responsibility…why do you always make me waste my damn time on your stupid school things?* (I would later come to realize that my dad, too, is human and is not immune to his own mental health issues.) At the time, I spit it back: *I hate you! I wish you weren't my dad.*

I ended up finishing laughably in 23rd place. I lay in bed, an endless recorded loop of negative thoughts spinning around in my head. I feared what my peers thought of me, what my teachers thought of me, what my parents thought of me. The thoughts devolved into a completely unrelated stream of anxiety: *I should lose weight; I look ugly with glasses and braces; I am hopelessly bizarre, unlikeable, and unlovable. I deserve this, I deserve this, I deserve this*, I repeated over and over in my bed until I fell asleep. When I had anxious episodes like these, my mother (always inherently the kinder and more understanding one) would hold me in her arms. She would tell me how much she loved me and ask me if it really was that big of a deal that I hadn't done very well in an extracurricular competition. (So many of my adaptive behaviors, I attribute to her.) On these days, my father would snap remorsefully back into his paternal role: *Life is hard, kid. You can't spend your life feeling sad about it.* I always forgave him, falling back into the role of being his daughter.

My procrastination and anxiety continued to tangle and multiply, and my father's rage and disappointment inevitably followed.

Step 1: Come up with a crazy, over-the-top, creative idea for an assignment.

Step 2: Procrastinate until the last possible minute.

Step 3: Work through the night (all the while not telling your dad, because your dad, especially your dad, will never understand) and tap into that favorite friend—anxiety—to guide you to the finish line.

Ignore him screaming over you to go to sleep, to stop being so irresponsible, to stop being so useless. Ignore the anxiety that's shaking you from the inside out. Let it soak into your body. Absorb it. Internalize it. Utilize it. Fight with Dad. Forgive Dad.

It was the script of my childhood. It worked beautifully. The teachers loved whatever overwrought project I brought into class: a Valentine's Day mailbox shaped like a USPS mail truck with a functional cargo door; a working volcano, diorama, and poem for an assignment that was meant to be an essay on Pompeii; a fully illustrated comic book of original Greek Mythology for a unit on Oedipus Rex. The teachers showered me with As.

These patterns continued past grade school. Through high school, my anxiety propelled me to levels of higher and higher success: prestigious awards, scholarships, school acceptances, speeches. My father was immensely proud of me, and I clung to his infrequent words of praise. In a convoluted way, my achievement became the basis for much of our relationship during my teenage years. In middle and high school, I went through a glorified dark "phase" when I wore only black and wrote lists and poems about all of the things I hated about myself and my life. I would often spend my

Sundays lying in bed, too anxious to move or eat, staring at the ceiling, feeling the individual weight of each minute passing by, each unread email in my inbox. My anxiety was not just something I felt or experienced transiently. It was so much bigger than that. It was an integral and overwhelming part of my personality that I came to depend on to find the motivation to sign up for new opportunities, to meet deadlines, to react quickly to the increasing mountain of responsibility I was accruing. During the best times, it was a presence that lived inside me, nudging me along. During the worst, it was me.

I moved away to college, and the anxiety persisted. It became much easier to deal with because I didn't have to deal with my father's reactive anger. However, I dealt with it through new, maladaptive coping strategies: all-nighters, alcohol, unhealthy relationships, and attachments with men who could falsely inflate my self-esteem with kind words and empty actions. I didn't call my dad during the first three months of school.

Much later, as I reflect on the lifecycle of my anxiety, I realize how deeply normal it all felt to me at the time. Just as I'd adapted to a more difficult course load in engineering school or to living alone or to being in a relationship, I'd adapted to making room for the anxiety in my life, because of its chronicity. It wasn't until I went to a doctor for an unrelated medical visit during college and filled out a screening tool for anxiety called the "GAD-7" that I considered what was happening to me wasn't normal. Generalized Anxiety Disorder. I stared at the words until they started to blur.

Sometimes, things must get much worse before they improve. My junior year of college, I began to develop panic attacks; I developed a concurrent eating disorder; I drank heavily four nights out of the week. At this point, I barely spoke to my dad, seeing him only during holidays. These times would inevitably turn the clock back; our fights were horribly repetitive and would frequently dredge up old emotions. Finally, one day around New Year's, I called my mom, sobbing. The anxiety was so bad I couldn't handle it anymore. I didn't want to die, but I couldn't live like this.

My mom didn't know what this meant, but she knew I was in trouble. We talked about therapy. She also, of course, told my dad. He tried to help in the ways he could: motivational speeches and stories about his own childhood. But his brash, pull-yourself-up-by-your-bootstraps attitude fell flat. He had grown up in India, a place where these kinds of things were next to taboo; the right words to say were simply not in his vocabulary.

Luckily, thanks to my strong support systems, including my university and my friends who had struggled with depression and anxiety, I discovered resources such as therapy and psychiatric services. Medications helped quiet the negative cognitive loops in my head so I could create more adaptive thoughts. Therapy helped me find the right words to describe and address my emotions. I relapsed a few times. I started over. I was able to eventually restructure my thoughts; this helped me end my self-destructive behaviors. I learned to name the anxiety; it lost its all-consuming power.

My father and I have made progress over the course of years; our relationship continues to improve. As a child, I craved his support and love. Over time, this craving rotted into disappointment. Years of distance and improved self-esteem have helped me reconcile this disappointment. We talk on the phone and sometimes meet for lunch when he's in town. And while he still doesn't completely understand, he accepts that I take medication; he's even apologized for how hard he used to be on me. My relationship with achievement and disappointment is also healthier. It is not perfect, and I sometimes regress into my old self, into old patterns of self-loathing and destruction. Through psychiatric support and perhaps the grace of some god, I am doing really, really well.

It is for this reason that having psychiatry as my last clerkship of the year feels significant. I spend the mornings learning the medicine: the parts of the interview, the medications, the therapies. I spend the afternoons visiting with the kids, my patients. We discuss the strategies they learned that day and their goals for the next day. It feels important to identify and modify their risk factors, rattle off the various treatments, and help them name the impact of their conditions on their thoughts and emotions. In this space, they reclaim their power.

Some people—even the psychiatrists—on the team call Abby narcissistic. She is stubborn, a know-it-all, withdrawn. But it is impossible for me to not like her, maybe because I see glimpses of myself in her. We talk about how it feels to be a minority at an all-white school, and she opens up about how she feels conflicted about her identity. We talk about what it's like to have dads who can be jerks, about what it's like to pretend not to care for so long that it hurts. We talk about how it feels to be put down by them, how that rejection can impact us in ways we don't always notice. I tell her something that surprises me as I say it.

"At the end of the day, you don't have to live with your dad forever, but you do have to live with yourself forever, Abby."

I don't know if Abby's father will ever come around. I don't know if my dad ever will fully either. But I know she will get better. I have learned there is a rhythm to the child psychiatry ward—a satisfying pattern that enables me to conceptualize the course of a mental illness as clearly as I could that of any other illness. On Monday, we admit a suicidal kid. By Saturday, they're home. It doesn't happen every single time, but it happens more often than you would expect. In between are daily cognitive behavioral therapy groups, support groups, social work evaluations, educational evaluations, coping skills groups, family meetings, assessments of home environments, insurance struggles, medication adjustments and additions, individualized action plans to address future negative thoughts or suicidal ideation, and follow-up appointments with therapists and psychiatrists. In between these are moms bringing pizza and nail polish to their kids' rooms to re-establish normalcy, dozens of conversations between the families and our team, devastating relapses, and fathers confronting their own issues and biases. And in between these are the individual and private moments of anguish; the countless moments of self-doubt; the strength, the hope, the belief; and the slow, but certain, arc toward recovery.

My Moving Feet

Kathryn Brown

Running is the one thing I've been able to keep constant this year, full of changing schedules and changing teams. My feet pound the ground, and I have a rare moment to myself, to let my mind wander. My feet are used to pounding. They pound the sidewalks to and from the hospital early in the morning and late at night, occasionally on a lucky sunny afternoon. They pound the hospital hallways, up and down the stairs. It's ok; I like the motion. And this year if I'm sitting still it probably means I'm taking an exam, so I'd just as well be moving.

———————

"ROSE! ROSE, CAN YOU OPEN YOUR EYES?" I am on neurology, yelling at my patient, an elderly woman lying in bed, with fluffy white hair that sticks up chaotically. She does not open her eyes. Seizures brought her to the hospital, and my neurology team found the growing brain tumor that was causing them. We placed her on medications to stop the seizures, causing her to be sedated; this is why I have to yell at her every morning to see if she will respond. Rose looks like a human being, so I suppose she was one, once. But as we wean her meds and she fails to arouse, I lose hope of meeting her.

Then, on the day she is scheduled to go home, I walk into the room to find Rose sitting up, attempting to comb her hair.

"WHAT ARE YOU DOING?" I yell out of habit.

"Trying to clean up this mess," she says. "I wish I had a mirror." I look at her, surprised she is speaking.

"You're going home soon," I say, not yelling anymore. "Are you looking forward to it?"

"Oh yes," she says, "I'm going to watch movies."

I smile. "Are you going to see Wonder Woman?"

"You know," she says, pausing with the comb midway through her hair to look me in the eye. "I don't really like those types of movies. They aren't real. I like the kind with real life in them." And with that, her nurse wheels her away for a scan. I stand for a minute in her empty room, looking at the comb left on her windowsill, thinking about all the good and the bad that real life had given her.

This year is very different from the first two years of medical school, when I spent most of my time sitting still. Those years, I opened my brain wide, poured in a river of facts, and hoped they would all fit inside. This year, I wade through the mess of information I've packed in, trying to create order from the disarray. I am also interacting with patients on a regular basis for the first time. Compared to book learning, when I yearned to do something "real," my third year has so much reality that it borders on surreal.

The first patient I cared for who died was on labor and delivery. I watched her go into the operating room (OR) for a routine C-section, excited for her to finally meet her baby. Then we heard that something was going horribly wrong. The team worked to save her. Hours later they left the OR; there was nothing more they could do.

I worked through that whole day, just as the rest of the team outside that OR did, because there were other women who needed us. On my way home, I managed to make it to the elevator before beginning to cry. My feet carried me through that evening, as I ran hard by the river, trying to feel and not to feel, trying to make sense of things and not to think at all.

The next day we went back to work. I scrubbed into a C-section, where the medical student's job is simply to help hold open the incision. However, when the physician pulled this baby out, she reached across the table and placed the infant in my stunned arms. He was a big baby, heavy in my hands, warm, wet, and wriggling as he let out a cry. What was I supposed to do with him?! I was so surprised all I could do was look at him and laugh. It was a moment joyful and unexpected. I held him up over the dividing curtain between the mother's head and her open belly. "Congratulations!" I called, before handing the infant to a nurse waiting with a blanket.

It was only later, when I got home, that I recognized we had been in the same OR in which the woman had died the day before. The realization was equally stunning and strangely expected. In a hospital, each moment carries immense gravity, and each is unique in its circumstance. These moments slide around me, hard to make sense of. They are like fireflies, lit up and gone in an instant.

How is medical school?

"It's good," I say when people ask. "I'm enjoying seeing patients, but it sure is keeping me busy!" This is true, but laughably shallow. It's hard to go deeper. It's hard to explain the immense pressure to study and perform, the unpredictable, long hours, and the wild highs and lows that come with treating patients. I'm not sure I could explain the highs and lows if I tried; I scarcely allow myself to feel them much.

I don't have time to process things like that. My feet pound away, and the patients flash by.

———————

My feet are running again. Down stair after stair I go, charging into the emergency room with the pediatric surgery resident. We are coming to evaluate a baby, only three weeks old, but very sick. Baby Nora is gray, hardly moving, heart fluttering too fast. There is blood in her diaper. Her mother wraps her arms around herself, as if physically holding herself together. Nora's intestines have twisted around themselves, cutting off blood flow to the lower half. Nurses scuttle around us as the resident tells the mother, simply, that her baby needs to go to surgery immediately, that we may not be able to save her intestines, that we may not be able to save her.

"Stay with them!" the resident says as she runs off to prepare the OR. The nurses leave, too, and suddenly I am the only one in the room with a mother who has just heard that her baby, healthy only a day before, might die. Her arms slacken; the strength she has been holding begins to fail, and she turns toward me. No book or lecture could have prepared me for what to do in that moment. I hold her as she cries on my shoulder.

"You are in the right place," I say. "These surgeons deal with this every day, and they will fight for your daughter."

Soon I am in the OR, gowned and gloved, and we are looking inside Nora's tiny belly. We "run the bowel," going from one end to the other, hand over hand, until we find the twist. The surgeon untwists it, and we watch as the bowel, dark gray in color, slowly turns a dark pink—healthy and alive. Knots in my own stomach—that I hadn't known were there—unclench.

The next day, I peek into baby Nora's room. Her mother is laughing, sitting with her own mother as she holds her daughter. The picture they make is lovely, perfect. I pause to capture this moment, then walk in and give her mother a much happier hug than the day before.

"Thank you for everything," she says.

———

Third year has shown me that it takes a certain fearlessness to care for patients. It takes an ability to make decisions in the face of uncertainty, to receive trust with grace, to continue when everything is telling you that you can't. The residents work so hard under so much stress, yet they are doctors in force, managing long lists of patients. Meanwhile, my classmates and I fight to stay abreast of just two or three. How will I ever reach their level in the 18 short months before I have an MD after my name? I can only have faith that, like the students before me, I'll make it. I keep moving, reminding myself that a few miles each day add up to thousands over a lifetime.

———

I am on internal medicine. It is a brutal service; while on the inpatient teams, we work six days a week, every few days staying 11 or 12 hours as we admit new patients. I struggle to simultaneously bring my best in the hospital, study the immense volume of material, and maintain some sliver of anything "not medicine" in my life. Light is fading fast from the sky, but I squeeze in a run—the one non-medical thing I have been able to maintain, more because it is tied to some sort of survival instinct than because I truly feel I have the time to do so.

Through the wooded path I go, muscles loosening, mind beginning to wander. It lands on heavy topics. My team informed multiple patients of newly metastatic cancer that week, discharging them all to comfort care at home. It's made me deeply sad, I realize as I run, and I am surprised it has taken me all week to name the weighty knot deep in my chest as sadness. It is hard to take time to feel when you are forever moving.

After a while, I remember something I've known for a long time: our goal is not to "fix" patients, but to help them to live the best lives they can with the cards they have been dealt. In that light, transitioning our patients to hospice is no longer a decision riddled with despair. We had done right by them.

I emerge from the tree-lined trail to run by the lakeshore. The early evening sun, warm on my skin, sparkles off water rippling with the trails of several crew boats out to practice. I am startled to hear the sound of a fiddle and then a string bass and guitar. A bluegrass band is practicing in the pavilion. For once, I stop. Staring out at the water and boats, I listen to the music and the cicadas. It is peaceful. I miss this feeling, I realize, surprised to have lost it somewhere along the way. I sit still, letting it fill me up. I will need this later, I know. My feet will be moving again soon.

Becoming a Good Patient

Anonymous

"How do you think about mediastinal tumors?"

A question. Directed at me. From a kind and handsome young intern, trying to help. I looked back at him blankly. I honestly didn't think I had *ever* thought about chest tumors. He pulled up a chest CT scan to help illustrate what he was about to explain to me.

"OK, what's that?" he asked, the little arrow on the screen pointing to a dark circle in the middle of the picture. It looked like a black hole, almost too perfectly circular to be of biologic origin, in the middle of irregular, bumpy shapes.

It is a simple structure, basic anatomy. It does something important. But nothing came to me. I stared at the screen.

"It's OK," he said, "I'm not grading you."

He thinks I have a case of the nerves. Shy, maybe. I was thankful my cover was intact. *I have to talk to my doctors about this.*

———

We were seven months into our third-year clinical rotations. The word-finding difficulties had gotten worse. The fatigue had become overwhelming. At the end of the day, I would go home and collapse, not sure if I would make it in the next morning, not sure I would get out of bed. By the end of the week, I would be so tired I would fall apart, break down, tears streaming.

I can't do this! I just can't do this! I didn't know what would happen to me, and I couldn't figure out how to make it stop.

Sleep deprivation, unrelenting pressure to perform, and being stuck in a world that repeatedly made it clear I was not to expect nor demand equality—a perfect recipe for a nasty flare-up of that old, haunting Post-Traumatic Stress Disorder (PTSD). Ghosts I thought I had buried—intense anxiety, panic attacks, anger, violent nightmares. Yet nobody was to mention that diagnosis for months to come. My doctors were treating symptoms, hoping their meds would work. Unfortunately, it also turned out it was a bad year for asthma. With my immune system beaten down by stress and lack of sleep, I caught every cold, and they all went straight to my lungs, lasting longer than they should. Working to breathe added to the fatigue. The albuterol inhaler increased my panic attacks—not an unexpected side effect.

I saw my doctors. Three that week. The third solved my problem for me. One of the nine medications I had been prescribed many months ago, even at a low dose, had been heavily sedating. I stopped taking the drug. Over the next few days, the thick fog that had engulfed my mind for those last nine months cleared. I had my brain back! I started studying madly, cramming, even though I knew it was futile—I had lost too much time.

But wait…a side effect?! That was just a side effect?! I just lost nine months of my life—nine months of my medical training, to a side effect?! I should have been angry, but I laughed. Shit happens. The cause and effect might have been more obvious if it had not been one of so many medications.

I went out for a drink with friends that weekend for the first time in almost a year. I had become a hermit without noticing.

But the medications weren't finished with me yet. One morning, halfway through my surgery rotation, I went to meet the team at the operating room. I didn't recognize the attending. I was confused, but I figured I was just tired. I was definitely sleep-deprived. I scrubbed, gowned, and gloved. Shortly after the procedure started, the attending asked me to move around the table to help drive the camera. I turned to go, not seeing a cord directly in my path until it was across the front of my gown.

"Watch where you're going!" She snapped. The nurse helped me re-gown and glove.

"Something isn't right. This is not like me," I said, quietly. I was getting dizzy, starting to sweat under my gown. I continued to walk around the table.

"Watch out!" It was the anesthetist this time. "You just broke sterility again!"

"But I didn't touch anything," I replied.

"You dropped your hand! Keep your hands above your waist!" The attending sucked her teeth and sighed, "Be careful."

The resident shook his head in disgust. I could have excused myself then, but I was determined not to give in to their chastisement.

Fine. I'll drive your [expletive] camera. I bit my tongue and stood there silently for the rest of the case, holding the camera, sweating bullets under my gown, wondering if I would go down on top of the patient. Luckily, between the surgical mask, the cap, and the safety glasses, no one could see much of my face.

Later that night, I lay in the darkness of my room, my head spinning, vivid evil lashing out of the darkness, jeering, taunting. Luckily, a small part of my brain knew it wasn't real, knew it was the drugs— but the voices were drowning out what was left of rational. I prayed to all the gods I didn't believe in that I would go to sleep. Restless, tortured, wanting to scream, and just waiting for it to be over, when there is nothing you can do, it turns out that praying is an instinct.

And in the morning, I would have to shake it off like nothing happened and go back into the hospital with a smile on my face.

This time, it was withdrawal. The refills for one of those nine medications hadn't gone through, despite my efforts. I had run out. Surgery rotations boast notoriously long hours—in the hospital nearly 80 hours a week, plus study time. I eventually got the refills, but not without another hit to my grades and my confidence. Another wasted week.

———————

At the beginning of the clinical year, I prioritized showing up and not complaining, as we had been told to do. I threw myself in wholeheartedly. I didn't know how to manage illness on top of medical school, and I didn't anticipate the complications that were to affect me. I didn't have a plan. When things went wrong, I was blindsided, and I struggled to regain a sense of control.

Gradually over the course of the year, I learned how to be a better patient. I bought some of those medicine boxes with little plastic dividers—one box for each day of the week—carefully filling them up and arranging for refills on my day off. But there were more problems with trips to Urgent Care after hospital shifts. Another medication caused a drug-induced aseptic meningitis—a condition that mimics an infection of the tissues covering my brain and spinal cord. I realized I needed to re-prioritize. I started scheduling appointments with each of my doctors once a month, rather than waiting until something went wrong. I notified clerkship directors and attendings, offering to make up the time while hoping that they wouldn't actually require that of me.

———————

We are getting close to the end of our rotations now. I have had a few good weeks lately. I go to a lot of appointments. The medications are stable, their side effects tolerable for now. I am cautiously optimistic.

Realistically, though, third-year medical school rotations are competitive, and there is no time for illness or complications. I would be lying to say I am not scared about the damage all this has done to my transcript. I don't know how I am going to explain those grades next year, when applying for residency programs. For a long time, I couldn't think about that application process at all. When I did, panic would rise up in my chest, followed quickly by heartbreak and helplessness. I would have to excuse myself, close the door to my room, tears welling up. I would wait for the panic to subside, talking sense into myself, hoping the fears were unfounded. But the truth is, I won't get any points for being a good patient.

Maybe Medicine Was a Mistake

Trisha Paul

Tell me something you love.

I love warm chocolate chip cookies, straight out of the oven.

Thank you. Tell me something you love.

I love reminiscing. I love talking to strangers.

Thank you. Tell me something you love.

I love to read, to write, to dance. I don't know yet if I love medicine.

We were gathered in a ballroom, a group of doctors and dancers, to explore the art of medicine through movement. I sat cross-legged, looking into the eyes of a person I did not know, struggling to remember what to say after "*I love.*" It had become all too easy to think about the things I did *not* love. In fact, it was recently that I had first thought to myself that I hated the person medicine had made me become. So with each answer, I tried to reorient my brain; to move away from what I did not love; to consider a love of things; and move toward a love of feeling, of experiencing, of existing.

I appreciated the gratitude in the stranger's gaze, for responses beyond a simple "*Thank you*" were forbidden. This exercise about body language felt like a cheesy dating game, but there was undeniable intensity in being so vulnerable with someone so immediately.

My decision to pursue a career in medicine was years in the making, a carefully considered and well-thought-out choice. While my pre-medical courses occasionally made me question whether I had the intellect and stamina to become a physician, I was never wracked with the self-doubt that has pervaded my experiences in medical school. Although I have found that caring for patients is infinitely gratifying, I can't overlook my fear that what it takes to become a doctor will preclude me from becoming the physician I want to be.

I had no way of anticipating the demands of medical education. As a pre-med student, I envisioned a kind of medicine that was always centered around caring for our patients. However, it has been challenging to recognize, as a medical student, that the goals of medical education are not always concordant with optimal patient care.

It started with the realization that medical education is based on a premise of performance, or what sometimes felt like deceit to me. A few months into my third-year clerkships, I suddenly understood the importance of feigning confidence for the sake of gaining experience. This didn't help with the guilt that consumed me after doing a vaginorectal exam on an anesthetized gynecology patient, though. Nor did it stop me from doing the exam in the first place, for fear of never having another opportunity.

The daily grind of pre-rounding in the hospital was an exercise in redundancy, of questionable educational value to me and seemingly little benefit for my patients. "A hospital is not a hotel," I was told by those senior to me. Although I didn't think I would ever get used to waking people up in the wee hours of the morning, I adapted. That I didn't think to question the value of this practice until months later stunned me.

And then there was the way we talked to and about patients. On rounds, we talked about patients outside of their rooms, often saying things we would never dare say inside. Or worse, we would gather around a patient who was naked beneath a thin veil of gown and look down at him or her in bed, saying things that we knew the patient did not understand, and that we did not fully intend for the patient to understand. As we left the room, we'd make a few half-translated statements, almost as an afterthought, in the somewhat blasé tone that tells patients and families that this isn't the time or place to ask questions.

What terrified me about all of this was how so many aspects of medicine that at first seemed unsettling quickly became normal. It bothered me to realize how immune I became—never forgetting, but quickly accepting, that this is the way of medicine. My disillusionment with medicine was simultaneous with my acceptance of it; this is what disgusted me most.

During winter break, as my body soared along the Sri Lankan coastline, far away from the hospital, my mind wandered back to a time when a senior physician offered some advice.

"You have to interrupt people in order to help them. Time is precious and we all know there's not enough of it. You must interrupt people in order to do our job."

"But wait," I thought to myself, as I finally had a moment to challenge the memory of that physician's guidance, "What if I don't want that kind of job?"

Surprising myself with my own question, I found my mind and heart eager to tread further:

"Maybe medicine was a mistake."

Like a reflex, I pulled out my notebook. I wrote down the words, letting them slowly sink in as they materialized on the page. I took a deep breath and looked back out the window. My stomach felt queasy at the thought, but in this safe space miles away from the hospital, I was willing to entertain the uncomfortable idea just for a moment.

While I previously couldn't imagine doing anything else with my life other than being a doctor, I knew this was no longer true. I've fantasized about being a freelance writer who spends her day coffee-shopping. I've wondered whether an English PhD would have better satisfied my intellectual curiosities. Or perhaps a different role in healthcare, as a social worker or psychologist, would have enabled me to pay attention to the psychosocial aspects of health about which I care deeply, the ones that always seem of peripheral concern to physicians.

I never thought that medical school would cause me to question a profession I had so passionately believed was my calling. It was surprising to me that the thought of medicine as a mistake even crossed my mind. But this thought helped me notice the ways in which medicine had changed me. In fact, it was liberating—to realize I don't have to let myself be changed in these ways.

There are moments in medicine that have made me pause. When I watch physicians crouch down on their knees at bedsides, to truly look their patients in the eye. Or when a handshake requires not merely one but both hands to entirely encase that of a patient's. When a resident spends his Friday evening playing the piano in the hospital lobby for a dying man and his wife. What I have witnessed in these beautiful moments is sincerity: doctors and patients alike can be vulnerable and authentic with one another. These doctors, acting in these ways, encourage me to find a way to practice medicine as I am.

These beautiful moments stood in stark contrast to the other message conveyed by many doctors. Emotional distance, I was told, was paramount for personal well-being, for self-preservation and self-care, for survival. A physician once told me about how he becomes "an empathetic machine" when he walks into patient rooms, how emotionally connecting with his patients is a performance that he can simply turn on and turn off as needed.

That's not the kind of person I am. For me, it is not enough to go through the motions. The best way I know to cope with the emotional challenges of clinical medicine is by allowing myself to get close to my patients, to feel alongside them. When all else seems hopeless, supporting my patients in the simplest of ways has proven to be more healing than anything I have offered through modern medicine. A warm blanket, a refreshing glass of water, soft tissues. A gentle presence, an attentive ear, understanding eyes. I give myself fully to my patients, and it makes me feel as though I have something meaningful to offer.

When I offered to walk with my patient one day, she looked up at me and asked, "Can you do that?"

"Yes," I insisted to her and to myself. "Yes, I can."

We walked, she with her walker and me beside her, pulling her IV pole down the confined hallways of the oncology floor as we talked about springtime and her garden of peonies back home.

I once brought red-hot fireball candies to a patient eager to go home, a gentle incentive for him to be patient with our team as we treated his illness. His reputation of leaving against medical advice preceded him and, to be honest, he scared me at first. But I sat down with him while he ate his lunch one day.

"That looks good," I said, gesturing to his fruity drink. I was touched when this tough man generously made an orange-cranberry juice concoction—just like the one he was sipping—to share with me.

Then there was the thank-you card filled to the brim with handwritten gratitude I received a month after I had cared for a patient, which took me by surprise. This patient's kind gesture assured me that, somehow, I had done right by him. I had moved him just as he had moved me.

I will never forget these moments. But there are times when they become difficult to remember, when I find myself getting caught up in the less-than-beautiful things that happen in medicine, the things that I do not love, the things that make me not love who I am. I want to practice the kind of medicine I believe in, the kind that motivates me, energizes me, and fulfills me. My kind of medicine is not a performance; rather, it revolves around my patients as they are, with me as myself. There are aspects of who I am and what I cherish that I refuse to compromise for the sake of medicine. I know now that I do not have to make such a sacrifice.

I want to learn how to love medicine, and, I suspect, I will always be learning.

When I Cared for Don

E. Joseph Klein

When I first met Don, he was transferred to us from the psychiatry floor—an introduction that would send many internists running. But I wanted to become a psychiatrist. In other words, I ended up being asked to help care for any patient who had ever seen a psychiatrist or just seemed a little weird.

Don had initially been admitted for electroconvulsive therapy (ECT) for severe depression with psychosis; he had stopped eating due to unrealistic fears of illness. This reached a peak a few months earlier when he had lost his job after crashing his semi-truck. His depression worsened: he stopped eating entirely and spent his time in bed without energy or motivation to move.

He had tried and failed with many antidepressants and now needed ECT, and it was working. His sister and caretaker told me she hadn't heard him say more than three words at a time for months, and now he was calling her on the phone every other day and they were talking—full conversations. She was amazed, as she had nearly lost hope that his depression would ever resolve. ECT has a powerful stigma in popular culture, with images of patients being dragged, strapped to a bed, screaming, and getting zapped. This is unfortunate because evidence shows it is a highly effective and rapid treatment with minimal side effects for many psychiatric illnesses—especially for patients like Don.

About a month into his stay at the hospital, Don was found to have low blood potassium levels. The first thing to do when a patient has hypokalemia, or low blood potassium, is to get an EKG: is this affecting the heart? Before I met Don, I read his EKG. It was concerning for hypokalemia as well as a myocardial infarction, a heart attack. ECT works very well and has few contraindications; it can be used with nearly every patient, except one who is actively having a heart attack. Don's blood marker of cardiac damage was elevated to the smallest degree detectable, and in the context of his EKG, he likely had some damage to his heart. His ECT treatments were stopped, and he moved to our floor.

When I went to see Don, he looked sick. "Looking sick" is hard to describe until you've seen someone who truly looks sick. It's a gut feeling, a gestalt that physicians gain during their training after seeing patients that look sick but are stable, and patients that look stable but aren't. I still hadn't gained that gestalt, but even I could tell that Don looked *sick*.

When I shook his hand, it was cold, weak, skeletal. When I listened to his lungs, I felt every bony ridge of his scapula and every string of muscle in his shrunken shoulder. When I felt his abdomen, I saw his pelvis bursting out of his taut, tired skin. Although there was no sign that Don was in immediate danger, the resident and I felt uncomfortable leaving the room without doing a little more work than is standard.

As I got to know Don and his family better, I learned his issues with eating were not new. His sister told me he constantly counted calories, started fad diets, and obsessed over his weight for as long as she could remember. He had always been thin, and his doctors had recommended he gain weight for years, but he had never been diagnosed or treated for an eating disorder. Depression is now recognized as a common disease in the elderly, but eating disorders are still often assumed to be isolated to teenage girls. Though stigma against mental health has vastly improved in recent years, it is still widely prominent, particularly in older generations of patients and their doctors.

Don's sister said that since starting ECT, Don had become more talkative than the last several months of silent self-starvation. However, she felt his malnutrition and weight loss were under-addressed. She was upset, crying; she told me he was killing himself with starvation. Even if he denied intention, he was dying, she said.

I dug through his history, and it was true. Nearly every day he had turned down meals, and it was clear the staff had been frustrated with the effort and time it took to convince him to eat. I decided I would take care of it myself. When he refused food, he gave me many reasons: he couldn't swallow (he could), he had diarrhea (he didn't), he was too full (he wasn't). We received calls from Don's nurses when he started refusing medications. He needed to take potassium pills to correct his blood level, so I spent 20 minutes with him convincing him to take them. It worked, but it was exhausting.

A lot happens in a patient's day. Don underwent a stress test for his heart, took several dozens of pills, and underwent a swallow study that proved he could swallow. He was started and stopped on multiple types of antibiotics, and I convinced him to eat his pudding—twice.

Even with these small victories, Don was malnourished and wouldn't eat more than a few bites. The medical solution is to place a feeding tube up through his nose and down into his stomach. But when presented with this solution, Don reacted strongly, refusing it. It was already determined that he was unable to make medical decisions, as he didn't demonstrate an understanding that his refusal of the tube would kill him, a topic he was always pushing to the next day. I felt uneasy with his potential loss of autonomy, so I spent time convincing Don that the feeding tube was the best choice. I asked him if he wanted to die. He said only to stop the pain. I asked if he was trying to die. He said no. I asked if he realized he *was* dying. He said he wasn't sure. I told him if he truly didn't want to die, then he needed the tube. He reluctantly agreed. It was a small comfort, as he would have gotten one anyway if his sister approved, but at least it wasn't against his will. The tube was our only chance of keeping him from slowly dying from starvation or suicide—the word choice is a matter of semantics.

Don was absorbed in events that, on the larger scale, are minute. They occurred constantly, relentlessly, and he was powerless. Don experienced each personally, and he often told me how exhausted he was in the afternoon after refusing a test, because he was just so tired. I also became absorbed in Don's minutiae. I knew where he was, always. I knew the results of every test, scrolled through every scan. I knew how much of his dinner he ate and how many pills he refused. His sister knew my desk phone number, and I had met their mother. He was my patient, and for the first time I felt the responsibility that entails.

But the problem with a "rotation" in medical school is that we rotate out as quickly as we rotate in. After knowing Don for a week, my rotation ended and I moved to a different hospital. I couldn't see Don's chart anymore and could not follow his course from afar as I often do now after I form a connection with a patient.

On the first day of my next rotation, I saw the resident who also took care of Don. We had rotated onto the same floor. He pulled me aside in the hallway and told me he remembered how close I was with Don. He wanted me to know that Don had died. I asked how. He thought it was aspiration, but wasn't sure. Don choked.

I remembered when Don had trouble swallowing his pills and how he was afraid he would choke, even though the swallow study said he wouldn't. I remembered how I told him he needed a feeding tube and how he refused and refused until I spent hours talking about it with him; how I stood next to him while it was placed and how he gagged and spat as they failed three times before getting it down. I remembered the minutiae, the small things that happened each day that affected him far more than I will ever know. I wondered if at some point, in a single second, something went wrong, and then he died. And I wondered if something I had done led to that second.

I had seen patients die before. I had helped operate on a child who was clearly not going to survive. I had seen patients in the hospital the day before they died, and then a different patient in the same bed the day after. I had watched doctors tell patients that they weren't able to do anything further, that this was the end. But Don was different. Don was *my* patient—I knew everything about him, explained everything to him, learned so much from him. Until then, I had been around death, but I hadn't had one of *my* patients die.

Immediately after learning this, I felt guilt. If he died from aspiration, was the feeding tube a part of that? If I hadn't convinced him to accept the tube, would he still be dying, but still alive? If I had stopped his sister from giving him a French fry, would his airways have stayed clear? If I hadn't pushed him to take all those pills, would anyone have even known he could swallow?

I wondered who told his sister. She had been so encouraged by his improvement and expressed so much hope. I wondered how she handled it. I wondered how the doctor presented it to her; was the doctor thoughtful or careless?

I wondered if anyone understood that he didn't truly die from aspiration, but rather, he died from depression, from anorexia, from stigma.

I wondered, worried, imagined, and hoped he was treated well until the end, that his death was just and not simply due to a failure on my part or someone else's. And I wondered if he finally found the relief he hoped for when he told me he wished he could just die.

A few seconds after he told me of Don's death, the resident was working on admitting a new patient. I didn't know if he felt like I did. I didn't know if he wondered, too. But then I looked at the whiteboard on the wall and saw a new patient had been placed on my list. So I did my job: I looked up the new patient, pushing Don to the back of my mind, another emotion suppressed and another "learning experience" committed to memory.

For the next two weeks, Don became abstract. He became a learning tool for the treatment of hypokalemia, an organizer for the workup of chest pain, and a mnemonic for the symptoms of depression. He also became a talking point on my clinical evaluation—I got an excellent grade for reasoning with Don when others could not.

While Don became all those things in my memory and on my transcript, he stopped being human. I think I felt true empathy, or something close to it, when he was a person sitting in front of me, breathing, speaking. But I left before he died. Though I experienced the hospital with him, I didn't experience the hospital without him. I didn't feel the loss.

I often feel uncomfortable hearing doctors, further along in their training, tell stories of patients. Many use humor to cope, and others put up an emotional wall. I've felt baffled as to how they could be so insensitive, how they could say these things about someone they knew. It seemed they had forgotten empathy, or at least how to be civil.

Yet, when I needed to remember how to treat hypokalemia on my exam, I thought about Don. I quickly remembered the diagnoses and treatments, but I didn't picture his face because that would have been impractical during an exam; emotions are extraneous when we require efficiency. I realize now that these moments of detachment aggregate into callousness, the seeming absence of empathy despite a doctor's position of deep intimacy. I now understand this callousness is not the loss of caring, but rather a shelter from caring, because caring hurts. If we feel every patient's emotion and pain as they feel them—with unbridled empathy—we drown.

I've asked mentors I respect about this problem, and I have not yet heard the answer I want. I have been told to have compassion, not empathy; to take care of myself, and then others; that otherwise it's too much; and that one day I'll understand. Maybe I'm naïve in thinking there is a way to maintain the empathy that currently makes my long days worthwhile, and I'm simply setting myself up for failure. Or maybe I'll find the secret, be the first to reach a balance between empathy and stability, and fix the deep-seated issue that makes doctors so susceptible to callousness. But not now—another patient just arrived.

Two Stories

Mary Guan

I am strong, I am competent, I feel nothing.
I am strong, I am competent, I feel nothing.

I recited these sentences throughout my third year of medical school; with each new rotation, I did my best to pretend to know what I was doing. Although third year exhausted me mentally, I felt it did not exhaust me emotionally as much as it did many of my classmates. My feelings fluctuated minimally between two rigid, straight lines, with few ups and downs.

I rotated through the Critical Care Medicine Unit (CCMU) my fourth year as a sub-intern. The patients in the CCMU are the definition of the "sick" we learn in medical school, with a long-running list of medical diseases that preclude them from receiving surgery. In other words, they are "surgical disasters," "medical disasters," or a combination of both. We took care of a 27-year-old man with recurrent pneumonias and every day a new section of his lung would collapse. He had been in the unit for nearly two weeks by the time our team took over. We rounded on a 45-year-old father with Bactrim-induced liver failure. Bactrim is a common drug, used to treat urinary infections, and this side effect was something you read about in a textbook but never expect to see in person. We also cared for a 60-year-old woman with heart failure that was extremely difficult to control (a smidge too much fluid or too little fluid would tip her over the edge into an irregular heartbeat). I found myself fascinated by the complexity of these patients, eager to learn about both the patient and the disease process occurring inside the body.

In the CCMU, I experienced many firsts. It was the first time I helped shave a stubborn patient's beard so he could have a better seal with his sleeping mask. The first time I worked to transition patients to comfort care and talked with grieving family members. The first time I filled out death certificates under the guidance of my senior resident. One of the few times I performed multiple rounds of CPR on a dying patient. And there were more.

Emotions. That's where I was going.

Ms. Wang was not my patient. She had been admitted overnight, and our team was rounding on her the next morning. Before we reach her room, the attending blurts out, "I couldn't sleep the entire night. I was up worrying about Ms. Wang and how her night went. What can we do for her? Let's put our heads together and discuss her case."

The resident described how Ms. Wang had been transferred from the cancer patient floor for septic shock, a widespread infection causing organ failure. She had been diagnosed with lymphoma two months prior and was originally admitted to the hospital for a fever. At that time, the team tested her for various infections. She was diagnosed with an inactive form of tuberculosis and was started on treatment. While in the CCMU, she deteriorated, so we added new antibiotics, administered fluids, and maintained her blood pressure with dangerous drugs that had to be monitored by the second. However, she did not improve, and we wondered if she might have an infection hiding in her bowels or soft tissue. But imaging showed no localized pocket of infection or acute process in her body. Running out of medical options, we continued to cover her with antibiotics.

I peered into Ms. Wang's room. Because her last name was Chinese, I felt a kinship and, thus, wanted to observe and evaluate her with my own eyes. Gathered around Ms. Wang were maybe 15 people: family members, friends, and acquaintances from the community. A wrinkled old man was to the right of her; a lady with a furrowed brow to her left; pre-pubescent teenage boys were mumbling to each other in the corners, glancing between their phones and Ms. Wang. A man with a leather-bound book in his hand was speaking quietly to Ms. Wang. Perhaps a bible prayer? I heard soft chatter in Mandarin—a dialect I didn't recognize, perhaps a local one?

A couple more kids wandered in and out of the room, wearing t-shirts with "Huron High School" emblazoned on the back, similar shirts to the one my brother wore day in and day out, refusing to change it for lack of a better reason except, "I don't smell anything strange coming from it." I had seen these elderly faces someplace else too, these men and women with their tired eyes, wrinkled cheeks, and graying fly-aways all out of place. They might have known my maternal grandma, who had lived in senior housing in Ann Arbor, a social butterfly who sang traditional songs in choir Tuesday mornings and practiced Tai Chi Thursday evenings. They had likely interacted with Zhang *laoshi*, my "Medicine in Mandarin" teacher from my second year of medical school ("Laoshi" is Mandarin for "Teacher," thus translating to "Teacher Zhang"), who knew nearly all the Mandarin-speaking patients in the hospital. Overwhelmed, I sped to the next patient's room to catch up with the team, who were still musing over how best to approach Ms. Wang's lack of improvement overnight. We worried about how much longer she would survive, given her tenuous situation. Before I knew it, while standing in the circle of white coats, a sense of despair and grief enveloped me, extending from the tip of my toes to my scalp. I started to feel dizzy, lightheaded, as if I was about to faint. I blinked. It worked. It kept tears from falling.

I am strong, I am competent, I feel nothing.
I am strong, I am competent, I feel nothing.

127

My grandma on my dad's side lived in China and had just passed at the start of my CCMU rotation. She died of metastatic stomach cancer. In China, the relationship between patient and physician is different, and it is occasionally supplanted by the relationship of the family to the physician. This was the case for my grandma. My aunts and uncles did not want her to know about the severity of her illness or her prognosis. They wanted the doctor to tell her that the cause of her early satiety, of her weight loss, of her nausea and vomiting, was a horrible anemia. She believed she would die of anemia. What else could she hold onto? After all, the only therapy she was aware of was the blood transfusions: first monthly, then weekly, then daily.

Meanwhile, my family made their farewells. My dad visited China—as he does every couple months for business—but this time made a conscious decision to stop by my grandparents' home as well. He had asked me over the phone how long I thought grandma was going to live. I advised him to go back to Nanjing; you never really know. I urged him to give my grandma more autonomy. He argued that, in China, the family unit acts as the decision-maker and that my grandma would not want to know what was happening to her. I understood my dad's point of view, but a part of my Western-educated brain kept wondering, "What would my grandma want?"

I never saw my grandma after she was diagnosed with stomach cancer. In my head, she remained healthy, a spunky old woman unable to pronounce English words with more than one syllable, which meant my name, Mary, turned into "Mar" when she said it.

———————

After long deliberation, our attending talked to Ms. Wang's family about transitioning her to comfort care. She could have a simpler death, surrounded primarily by her community rather than superfluous medical equipment. Shortly after the family agreed to comfort care, Ms. Wang passed. Watching her die less than 24 hours after being admitted to the CCMU made me contemplate. Had my grandma been surrounded by a gathering of family and friends? Had anyone prayed for her during those last hours? My grandma had never known the cause of her death. Neither had Ms. Wang. She had had septic shock, but what caused it? Both elderly women were unlucky to have been diagnosed with metastatic cancer. Although both may have died with peace of mind, neither had died knowing exactly why. I reminded myself that the reason for a patient's death is something we, in medicine, like to know for our own sanity, but it's not something patients need or necessarily want to know.

Ms. Wang had diffuse bowel edema, giving her something we call "abdominal compartment syndrome," in which the pressures inside her abdomen were so high her bowel probably just burst. That was what the autopsy findings said.

I am strong, I am competent, I feel... ruined, like the charred remains of burrowed termites after a forest fire.

The tsunami-like intensity of the CCMU had crashed into me, knocked me over, and left me with bruises and scrapes no other rotation had been able to deliver. Nevertheless, I am glad for having experienced the blows. As inhuman and terrible as I felt while a third-year student, I was nevertheless a human being, replete with sadness, anger, fear, and happiness. Now, when my late grandma enters my thoughts, as if on cue, the memory of seeing Ms. Wang's entire community stuffed into one room appears simultaneously. I feel the urge to comfort her grandchildren and her loved ones and pray alongside them; yet I am mournful for the impact her loss will bring on her family. These feelings engulf me, saturating my consciousness. Eventually, I willingly tire out and accept my own emotions with relief.

Yes, I Understand

Sara McLaughlin

It was a hot summer day in early August. I gathered with 170 strangers and their families for the White Coat Ceremony to celebrate our entry into medical school and the start of our medical careers. Like most of my soon-to-be classmates, I was full of excitement and anticipation. I had been accepted to the medical school of my dreams to pursue my dream career. I had returned to my hometown, which I had loved and missed. Unbeknownst to my peers, I was on the verge of becoming more than a medical student; I was 10 weeks pregnant with my first, much desired pregnancy. I looked around: Who would become my closest friends? Who would I tell first? How long did I have to wait to share my good news?

We began medical school studying Genetics. It seemed as if each lecture was directed at me and my growing belly. When we learned about rates of trisomy 21, I wondered if my baby was carrying extra chromosomes. A woman spoke to us about her decision to continue her pregnancy even though the baby likely had Down Syndrome. We met her son and heard about his successes and struggles. "I just want him to find love someday," his mom said, to a hall of damp eyes. I had no idea what I would do if the results of my genetic testing came back with news similar to hers. The year continued. I made friends. I held on to my secret.

And then the day I will never forget: August 22, my first obstetric ultrasound. Baby pops up on the screen. Bright, smooth ribs and spine, evenly spaced in geometric perfection. Limbs moving. So human. A flawless baby, like ultrasound images I had seen from friends and would come to study in the years ahead. The ultrasound technician leaves the room, and a physician enters. The appointment, which was supposed to be a joyous confirmation of the baby to come, instead becomes a blur of badness.

"We don't see a uterus."

"Possibly ectopic."

The pregnancy was so far along, already 13 weeks. A ticking time-bomb. I step back and wish with all my might that this isn't happening, but I cannot stop time or change the course of fate.

"No, you can't fly to your cousin's wedding. You need to go to the Emergency Department (ED), right now. I'm sorry."

Hours later, an MRI and more ultrasounds. I email professors and classmates from my bed in the ED with vague reasons for missing meetings and assignments. I'm sent home in a daze. More diagnostic studies, more conversations, more wondering if my baby would live. More attending class and taking quizzes as if life were normal. One week later, the final verdict: a rare uterine anomaly, the doctor told me, a bicornuate uterus with one rudimentary horn, unfit to hold a pregnancy but with one growing inside. A uterine horn that almost certainly would rupture should I continue the pregnancy. So the pregnancy had to end, or my own life would be in serious danger. My rational nature and budding medical knowledge evaporated. It was all my fault. The floor dropped out from under me. My perfect baby had to die because of my horribly imperfect body. Nothing could make me feel that this wasn't my fault. I sobbed and apologized over and over to my baby.

That fall, in Doctoring class, we discuss how to deliver bad news, to consider how the news might affect a patient. We talk about how, for a patient, bad news may split life into "Before" and "After." Yes, I understand. I was living After and could never return to Before.

Then came the worst day of my life: the day we had to end the baby's life. Potassium chloride injection into the little heart. Heart stops, and the worst cramps I'd ever felt start. I pick my head up, walk from the clinic to the library, and sit in front of a computer screen in a fruitless attempt to study. My husband drives me home. I assume the fetal position. I cry and cry. Then I finish studying and take an exam in a parallel universe where life is okay. Weeks later, while studying the cardiovascular system, I learn how hyperkalemia, too much potassium, can cause the heart to beat abnormally or even stop. I become nauseated. Yes, I understand.

Next came surgery. Removal of the faulty uterine horn and its contents. I wake up. My shoulder hurts. In anatomy, I learn that the diaphragm is controlled by the same nerves that go to the shoulder, often causing shoulder pain with diaphragm irritation. Yes, I understand. My physical pain is severe, much worse than I had expected. Emotional pain can cause or augment physical pain, I learn later. Yes, I understand.

In Doctoring class, I learn about being an empathic physician who supports patients' emotional and physical well-being. I walk, from a morning of pretend examples and role-play, to my doctor's office, where he puts a hand on my knee and looks me in the eye.

"We've been talking a lot about how you've been doing physically; how are you doing up here?" he asks, pointing to his head.

I break down.

He says, "This and that might be hard."

I don't remember what his "this and that" were, but I remember he was exactly right. I hadn't said it, for it was too hard to say. But he knew. With a warm embrace, my tears began. I looked up and thanked him for making me, the patient, feel like it was going to be okay. At the same time, I thanked him for giving me, the medical student, a perfect example of the empathy and caring I would attempt to emulate for the rest of my career.

During the second year of medical school we learned about pathology—what can go wrong. My second year was accompanied by two more pregnancies. I was a nervous mess the whole time. In class we learned about early pregnancy problems—abortions, they're called—of all types. Pregnancy number two ended in a spontaneous abortion, or miscarriage. With the third pregnancy, I experienced a threatened abortion: fifty percent chance of the pregnancy continuing. A jarring statistic. Yes. I understand. Somehow, I was dealt the lucky cards and the pregnancy marched ahead.

Trisomies: The first trimester screen showed an increased chance of trisomy 18. Later, during my Pediatrics rotation, when I helped take care of a baby with trisomy 18, I could barely enter his room without feeling nauseated and weak in the knees. His less-than-one-year life expectancy, his microcephaly—or abnormally small head—and all of his physical difficulties...I was overwhelmed by how all of this must pain his parents. And I was filled with emotions as if he were my child. As I stood in the boy's room, I was unable to look him or his family in the eye. I felt powerless to this extra chromosome. Follow-up testing of my pregnancy showed no extra chromosomes. I breathed a sigh of relief. Time moved onward.

My half-sized, abnormally shaped uterus continued to expand and support my baby. He became too big to view in one screen on ultrasound.

He kicked me.

I told people.

I began to let myself hope.

I took Step 1 of the U.S. Medical Licensing Examination. I entered the wards.

And then a miracle: my beautiful and perfectly healthy baby boy was born. Another dividing line, another Before to After. A line I had come to believe I would never get to cross. I was a mom.

Now, I am an almost-physician with a toddler running around my home. My medical knowledge has expanded exponentially. I feel ready to have two extra letters affixed to my name and to claim all the responsibilities that come with them. I am a mom, and my life is full of love, amazement, and satisfaction (as well as dirty diapers and sleepless nights). The despair I have experienced along the way, however, continues to remain tangible. I remember the importance of empathy and seemingly simple acts, like a hug or check-in note. I remember how personal medicine can be. What an honor it is to care for others' bodies and souls. Yes, I understand the importance of this work and how difficult it can be both for patient and provider. I graduate prepared to tackle this daunting task, thanks to my infinitely entwined journeys as both a student and a patient of medicine.

On Becoming a Surgeon

Katherine Bakke

On a Sunday night in November, during our first year of medical school, my roommate and I sat at our kitchen table and decided to predict the future. With a list of the 170 people in our matriculating class in front of us, we attempted to guess which specialty each of our classmates would enter in four years.

For Alex, a quiet man who loved his grandmother, we chose geriatrics.

For Chris, a guy who always made slightly inappropriate jokes, we chose urology. (Only later did we learn that both his father and two brothers were urologists; we knew then that our prediction, and Chris' fate, was sealed.)

For Monica, an outspoken feminist, we chose OB/GYN.

When we came to my name, my roommate looked at me expectantly. "Well," she said. "What about you?"

She and I had met only three months before and were still getting to know one another. We had yet to talk about why we wanted to become doctors, about what experiences had motivated us to choose this path.

For me, there was only one answer. "I want to be a family doc," I said. "I'm sure of it."

As a senior at a Catholic high school, I first started entertaining the idea of becoming a doctor. My theology classes had a surprisingly progressive bent, and I admired modern-day saints like Dorothy Day and Thomas Merton for their bone-deep commitment to serving others. Upon graduation, I believed that the world would be a better place if people simply remembered their responsibility to others, and I was intent on leading a life in that manner. This moral conviction was with me when I entered college and carried me through four years of pre-med courses. It also gave me the sense that becoming someone's primary care physician was the purest moral pursuit in medicine.

Which was why, halfway through my third year of medical school, I faced an identity crisis. I wanted to be a surgeon, I had realized, and it felt like a shameful secret. I had predicted my future incorrectly. No one likes to be wrong when they were so certain they were right.

I never thought I wanted to be a surgeon. The depictions I saw on television, the jokes I heard in medical school, and the stories my physician father and nurse mother told me all depicted surgeons as heartless and unfeeling, arrogant and selfish. Worst of all, they hated patients—and I didn't want to be a doctor like that.

Yet, my surgery rotation had proven these myths wrong. Aside from finding surgical pathology interesting and working with my hands immensely satisfying, I was drawn to surgeons because they stand on the precipice of hubris and humility. The very nature of their jobs—cutting people open with only an inkling of what they might find inside—required an outrageous degree of confidence. But they also had a profound sense of humility. Despite the sophisticated operations and medicines they used to keep their patients alive, what they were really offering was time for the body to heal. Sometimes, the body could not heal, in which case, they offered up compassion to their dying patients and their families fiercely, sincerely. Their sense of responsibility to their patients astounded me and resonated with the moral convictions that had led me to medicine in the first place.

My interest in medicine, from the very beginning, had nothing to do with science and everything to do with people. People are peculiar, and contradictory, and they have this incredible capacity to withstand hardship and offer up love. I wanted to be with people, and serve them, in their most vulnerable times. I wanted to be the doctor who loved her patients, not despised them. It took me a long time—over a year—to understand that I could be a surgeon who loved her patients just as well as I could be a primary care doctor who did the same. Once I realized this, I knew it was the right decision. I was going to be a surgeon. I was sure of it.

———————

Everyone else, however, wasn't. Surgeons and physicians in other specialties looked at me with skepticism when I told them I was going to be a general surgeon. Seemingly everything about me—from my bubbly personality to my interest in health disparities to my curly hair—gave people a reason to question my decision. Throughout my fourth year of medical school, I heard:

"You're too nice to be a surgeon."

"Do you want to be miserable for the rest of your life?"

"If you're going to be a surgeon, you need to be more aggressive."

"You radiate empathy, but to be a surgeon you need to be tough."

"Do you want to get married and have kids?"

"That you occasionally get tired at work makes me think you can't hack it."

"I feel sorry for you."

"You should probably just do quality improvement projects instead of health disparities research."

"You should train in a big city so you can find a man who won't be intimidated by an ambitious woman."

"Are you *sure* you want to be a surgeon? You should think harder about it."

"Do you hate yourself? The training is brutal."

"Make sure you look nice on your interviews; people will think your curly hair is unprofessional."

"Do you have an exit strategy?"

"A career in surgery will be wasted on you."

Fourth year of medical school is supposed to be exciting, a time where one is supported and encouraged to realize their dream. Yet, I felt anything but. The persistent comments sent me a clear message: You don't fit in, you don't belong, this isn't for you.

When I met with one of the medical school deans to discuss my residency application, I burst into tears when she asked me, kindly, to tell her why I wanted to be a surgeon. For months I had tried to downplay the comments, rationalizing that they stemmed from one person's bad experience working with a surgeon, or were well-intentioned but poorly expressed concerns about being a woman in a traditionally male profession. But it didn't matter. It all felt extremely personal. To become a surgeon had not been an easy decision for me to make, and now I feared I would be an outsider in whatever residency program I matched. My concerns about fitting in felt both childish and very, very human.

She handed me a tissue, and I managed to make it through the rest of the meeting. But afterwards, I left her office and cried from humiliation and insecurity. It wasn't the last time.

That fall, I watched my friends receive numerous interview invitations to prestigious surgical programs while I took any interview I could get, be it in Omaha, Nebraska or Worcester, Massachusetts. That Hopkins or Brigham declined to interview me within a few weeks after submitting my application reinforced my insecurity that I didn't fit the typical mold.

I sat through three months of interviews noticing surgeons noticing me: the run in my nylons, the absence of a wedding band on my left hand, my curly hair, the fact that my CV suggested I should be anything but a surgeon. I also noticed that, while shaking more than one surgeon's hand upon the close of an interview, they looked me in the eye and smiled—surprised—and thanked me for an engaging conversation. Being different had its advantages, I learned, one of which was the ability to defy expectations in a memorable way.

In March, after nearly a year of self-doubt, I matched into my top-ranked general surgery residency program. I believed it was a place where I could be myself, which was why I placed the program at the top of my list, well ahead of other programs that had more money, more resources, and more prestige. I was thrilled, upon opening my envelope, to know they wanted me for who I am.

Medicine is a culture, and as such, comes with its own identity politics. Choosing one's specialty is not so much professional as it is a deeply personal decision. My third year of medical school was incredible, in part, because I had never learned so much about myself in such a concentrated period of time. These discoveries were something neither I nor my roommate could have predicted on that Sunday in November, our first year of medical school. After all, I was not alone in this: Alex, who still loves his grandmother, became an

anesthesiologist. Chris, by destiny, a urologist. Monica, like me, surprised herself during her third year and went on to train in pediatrics.

The ethos of general surgery resonated with my core values and
it was this, above all else, that attracted me to the field. Yet, to have
both surgeons and non-surgeons alike make me feel as if I did not
belong engendered a profound self-doubt that I carried with me until
the day I matched.

The hospital is a noisy place, full of alarms and beeps and phones
that ring. It is also full of voices, some of which offer encouragement
and others that do not. The latter are usually louder, although occasionally the former break through the din, and clearly.

I credit my medical school classmates, who remarked that I was
the most enthusiastic and energized when on my surgery rotation,
for being the first people to validate my decision.

I credit my lifelong friends, who jumped up from their seats in
celebration when I told them I was going to be a surgeon, for helping
me see past the criticism of others.

I credit my father—an internist—for realizing that surgery was
the best path for me, and my mother—a nurse—for saying, "You can
do it, Kerri!" in her best Bela Karolyi voice every time I called home
discouraged.

And I credit the doctors who punctuated their stereotyped
remarks about surgeons with a glimmering asterisk, a hopeful post-
script: "You know, surgery needs people like you."

———————

A few weeks after I matched, I cracked opened a fortune cookie at
the end of a Chinese take-out dinner I had shared with some medical
school friends. My fortune read: "It's kind of fun to do the impossible."

A friend sitting next to me leaned over to read the tiny slip of paper I held in my hand.

"That's perfect for you," she said, and I smiled.

About the Writers

Anonymous cares deeply about the so-called Social Determinants of Medicine, and she believes that promoting health means removing social and environmental barriers to healthy living. She has aspirations of spending her career promoting women's health and reducing barriers to care for all disadvantaged populations.

Katherine Bakke is a graduate of both the University of Michigan Medical School and the Harvard T. H. Chan School of Public Health. She currently lives in Worcester, MA, and is a general surgery resident at the University of Massachusetts.

Kathryn Brown is a medical student at the University of Michigan Medical School who is passionate about women's health, reproductive justice, and finding the humanities in medicine. When not at the hospital, you'll probably find her running along the Huron River or puzzling over the *New York Times* Sunday crossword.

Hailing from Southern California, **Jack Buchanan** meandered to medical school by way of Wisconsin, where he completed graduate studies in agriculture, environment, and philosophy. He hopes to one day marry his lingering interests in ethics and metaphysics with an actual career, probably in psychiatry.

Hannah Cheriyan is a student in the Medical Scientist Training Program (MD/PhD) at the University of Michigan Medical School, completing her PhD in Cancer Biology. She is so thankful to God for having the privilege of learning to care for patients, and she hopes to use her passions for research, patient care, and writing to change the world for the better.

Apoorv Dhir was born and raised in the best city in the world (Pittsburgh, PA) and is thrilled to be a part of this project. Outside of writing and medicine, Apoorv is an avid musician and enjoys singing and making music with friends in his spare time.

Mary Guan is a fourth-year medical student whose interests include cancer biology, eating various forms of carbs, and reading indie music blogs.

Meredith Hickson is in her final year of medical school at the University of Michigan, and she plans to pursue a career that combines pediatrics and global health. She has worked on various public health and research projects in sub-Saharan Africa since 2011.

Hadrian Kinnear is an MD/PhD student at the University of Michigan. He is interested in reproductive science/medicine and LGBTQ health.

E. Joseph Klein grew up in Michigan and plans to become a psychiatrist with a passion for mental health, stigma, and physician-patient communication. He spends his time playing music and exploring the outdoors.

Hsin (Cindy) Lee is a fourth-year medical student going into obstetrics & gynecology. Besides sharing and processing experiences through writing and coffee shop chats, she gets particularly lively when talking about favorite books, dance, her little sister, and food (especially Chipotle).

Sara McLaughlin is a resident physician in pediatrics at the University of Michigan. She lives in Ann Arbor, MI, with her husband and two-year-old son.

Anitha Menon is first, a lover of the arts and second, a lover of the sciences. She grew up reading anything she could get her hands on at the library and writing poetry. When she's not in the hospital, you can find her outside: backpacking, hiking, or exploring.

Originally from Idaho, **Daniel Nelson** plans to become an academic general internist and perform research in health policy. His other interests are largely limited to his wife and two children, who are wonderful—but occasionally he finds time to read a book or eat brownie ice cream.

Trisha Paul is a soon-to-be graduate of the University of Michigan Medical School who is excited to begin her training in pediatrics. She aspires to be a pediatric oncologist and palliative care physician, and she is passionate about ethics, narrative medicine, dancing barefoot, and buying anything made of cork.

Hanna Saltzman is a second-year medical student at the University of Michigan. Prior to medical school, she studied anthropology at Williams College and worked for environmental and public health non-profit organizations.

Mason Shaner is a first-year student at the University of Michigan Medical School and a former inner-city high school teacher with a background in biomedical engineering, stem cell research, and music composition. Her native Southern California spirit enjoys the genuine seasons of Ann Arbor and now appreciates that football is more than a sport.

Gabrielle Shaughness is a dog-lover who spends her free time taking long walks through wooded paths or enjoying the fellowship of her church community. Her favorite place to sit and read is on a Southern porch, where she has passed entire days in complete contentment.

Erika Steensma is a second-year medical student interested in studying geriatrics. In her free time, she enjoys running, baking, and reading.

Anita Vasudevan is a second-year medical student with an interest in primary care and integrative medicine. She enjoys cooking and practicing yoga, and she hopes to center her future clinical practice around the values that drew her to the medical field.

Nithya Vijayakumar grew up in Michigan and is interested in working to address and improve health disparities. She also enjoys martial arts, popcorn, and poetry.

Anonymous wrote most of her piece as a journal entry while she was a second-year medical student and found converting it to a (semi-) polished form to be both cathartic and healing. Having now completed her third year of medical school, she is strongly considering psychiatry as a future specialty. So it goes.

About the Editors

Trisha Paul (*Editor-in-Chief*) is a soon-to-be graduate of the University of Michigan Medical School who is excited to begin her training in pediatrics. She aspires to be a pediatric oncologist and palliative care physician, and she is passionate about ethics, narrative medicine, dancing barefoot, and buying anything made of cork.

Katherine Bakke (*Senior Editor*) is a graduate of both the University of Michigan Medical School and the Harvard T. H. Chan School of Public Health. She currently lives in Worcester, MA, and is a general surgery resident at the University of Massachusetts.

Whit Froehlich (*Senior Editor*) is an Ann Arbor native who holds a degree in Mathematics and Economics from Amherst College. He appreciated the privilege of working with his fellow medical students to share their stories about the unique experience of medical school.

Samantha Chao is a newly minted clinical student at the University of Michigan Medical School. She graduated from Carleton College in 2016 where she was an English and Chemistry major.

Alissa Wall Kleinhenz is a third-year medical student who studied contemporary American literature and cellular biology as an undergraduate. In her free time, she enjoys hiking, snuggling with her cat, and re-reading *All the King's Men*.

Anitha Menon is first, a lover of the arts and second, a lover of the sciences. She grew up reading anything she could get her hands on at the library and writing poetry. When she's not in the hospital, you can find her outside: backpacking, hiking, or exploring.

Rasna Neelam loves studio art, telling stories, re-watching old *Saturday Night Live* videos, avoiding studying, and anything related to the humanities. She is a second-year medical student at the University of Michigan, hoping to become a pediatrician and children's author in the future.

Hanna Saltzman is a second-year medical student at the University of Michigan. Prior to medical school, she studied anthropology at Williams College and worked for environmental and public health nonprofit organizations.

Julia Schoen is a fourth-year medical student at the University of Michigan who is going into radiology. Narrative writing and editing *iatrogenesis* provided an important creative outlet and community for her in medical school.

Jennifer Sun is an MD/PhD student at the University of Michigan Medical School who recently returned to the wards after completing her PhD in Developmental Psychology. She is interested in pursuing a career in primary care with a focus on psychosocial determinants of health. In her free time, she enjoys dancing, traveling, and baking French pastries.

Gina Yu is a second-year medical student at the University of Michigan who attended college at Harvard University, where she wrote for the Harvard Crimson as an editorial columnist and served on the editorial board. She has found working as an editor for this book very rewarding, and she values personal reflection through narratives in medicine.

CPSIA information can be obtained
at www.ICGtesting.com
Printed in the USA
BVHW04s2121020918
526198BV00006B/21/P